COPING WITH BREAST CANCER

Dr Eadie Heyderman, who herself had breast cancer, was a consultant pathologist and directed a research laboratory concerned with cancer diagnosis at St Thomas's Hospital, UMDS, London. She qualified at University College Hospital and is now Emeritus Reader in Histopathology in the University of London. She is married and has two sons, two daughters and one grand-daughter

D1630420

Overcoming Common Problems Series

For a full list of titles please contact
Sheldon Press, Marylebone Road, London NW1 4DU

The Assertiveness Workbook
A plan for busy women
JOANNA GUTMANN

Beating the Comfort Trap
DR WINDY DRYDEN AND JACK
GORDON

Birth Over Thirty Five
SHEILA KITZINGER

Body Language
How to read others' thoughts by their
gestures
ALLAN PEASE

Body Language in Relationships
DAVID COHEN

Calm Down
How to cope with frustration and anger
DR PAUL HAUCK

Cancer – A Family Affair
NEVILLE SHONE

Comfort for Depression
JANET HORWOOD

Coping Successfully with Hayfever
DR ROBERT YOUNGSON

Coping Successfully with Migraine
SUE DYSON

Coping Successfully with Pain
NEVILLE SHONE

Coping Successfully with PMS
KAREN EVENNETT

Coping Successfully with Panic Attacks
SHIRLEY TRICKETT

**Coping Successfully with Prostate
Problems**
ROSY REYNOLDS

**Coping Successfully with Your
Hyperactive Child**
DR PAUL CARSON

**Coping Successfully with Your Irritable
Bowel**
ROSEMARY NICOL

**Coping Successfully with Your Second
Child**
FIONA MARSHALL

Coping with Anxiety and Depression
SHIRLEY TRICKETT

Coping with Blushing
DR ROBERT EDELMANN

Coping with Bronchitis and Emphysema
DR TOM SMITH

Coping with Candida
SHIRLEY TRICKETT

Coping with Chronic Fatigue
TRUDIE CHALDER

Coping with Cot Death
SARAH MURPHY

Coping with Crushes
ANITA NAIK

Coping with Cystitis
CAROLINE CLAYTON

Coping with Depression and Elation
DR PATRICK McKEON

Coping with Postnatal Depression
FIONA MARSHALL

Coping with Psoriasis
PROFESSOR RONALD MARKS

Coping with Schizophrenia
DR STEVEN JONES AND DR FRANK
TALLIS

Coping with Strokes
DR TOM SMITH

Coping with Suicide
DR DONALD SCOTT

Coping with Thyroid Problems
DR JOAN GOMEZ

Coping with Thrush
CAROLINE CLAYTON

Curing Arthritis Exercise Book
MARGARET HILLS AND JANET
HORWOOD

Curing Arthritis Diet Book
MARGARET HILLS

Curing Arthritis – The Drug-Free Way
MARGARET HILLS

Overcoming Common Problems Series

Overcoming Common Problems Series

Overcoming Common Problems

COPING WITH
BREAST CANCER

Dr Eadie Heyderman

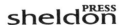
sheldon **PRESS**

First published in Great Britain in 1996 by
Sheldon Press, SPCK,
Marylebone Road,
London NW1 4DU

British Library Cataloguing-in-Publication Data
A catalogue record for this book is available from the British Library
ISBN 0–85969–726–6

Photoset by Deltatype Ltd, Ellesmere Port, Cheshire
Printed and bound by J. W. Arrowsmith Ltd, Bristol

Acknowledgements

Sources of the information used in this book

The information and statistics used in this book are drawn from a number of sources and I am grateful to have been able to use them. The most important are:

De Moulin, D., *A Short History of Breast Cancer*, Martinus Nijhoff Publishers, 1983.

Whelan, S. L., Parkin, D. M., Masuyer, E. *Patterns of Cancer in Five Continents*. World Health Organisation Publication, IARC Scientific Publications No. 102, 1990.

Cancer Statistics Registrations MB series and Mortality Statistics Cause DH Series for England and Wales, Office of Population, Consensus and Surveys, HMSO, 1971 onwards.

Cancer Research Campaign Factsheets, Cancer Research Campaign, 1988 onwards

Ethnicity and Health, Department of Health, 1993.

The Health of the Nation and The Health of the Nation One Year On, Department of Health 1992 and 1993

Social Trends 1995 Edition, Central Statistical Office, HMSO, 1995.

Trademarks

The following trademarks are mentioned in the book:
Adriamycin (Doxorubicin) was a registered trademark of Pharmacia Ltd.
Lentaron (Formestane) is a registered trademark of CIBA Laboratories
Zoladex (Goserelin) is a registered trademark of Zeneca Pharma

Contents

Introduction

Your problem is mine

I had surgery and radiotherapy for breast cancer in 1991 when I was 59. At the time, I was a consultant pathologist and directed a research laboratory concerned with cancer diagnosis. I am not sure whether it's better or worse to be 'in the trade' when something like this happens: I was only too aware of everything that could go wrong, all the possible complications. Although I was pretty certain of the diagnosis, it was still devastating to have it confirmed. Like most women I thought, 'Why me?', and 'I don't want to die'. I looked enviously at other women on my way home. Why were they so healthy and full of life when I had this thing growing in my breast? The surgeon who made the diagnosis and later carried out my operation was a colleague and a friend. I managed to stop myself from crying when he told me he thought the lump was probably malignant. When I got home I collapsed into tears.

In some ways it was much easier for me as a doctor, familiar with hospitals and medical jargon, but in many ways it was more difficult. I always felt that, even more than other women, I had to put a brave face on things and 'be good'. As a pathologist, part of whose job it was to investigate the cause of death in cancer patients, my main experience of women with breast cancer was of those who had died. It was not until I had cancer myself, and talked to friends and neighbours about it, that I became aware of the many women who were alive and well many years after their treatment. Cancer of the breast has almost the highest survival rate of cancers in adult women. 62% of women with breast cancer are still alive after five years – a percentage which is only bettered by cancer of the uterus, with a 70% five-year survival, and cancer of the thyroid with a 65% 5-year survival in women (five years is taken as an achievable time to follow up patients, since they may change their address and be difficult to trace after five years). This compares well with the 8% five-year survival for lung cancer and under 4% for cancer of the pancreas.

My cancer was small. I was treated by lumpectomy (removal of the cancer) and axillary clearance (removal of the lymph glands in my armpit), followed by radiotherapy. Survival is not necessarily the same as cure, and some of us will have a recurrence later. Much of the time, women with breast cancer feel there is a Sword of Damocles hanging over their heads. I try not to let my cancer overshadow my life but none the less, if I have any unusual symptoms, I think my cancer has recurred – a headache, for example, immediately makes me think that cancer has spread to my brain. I started swimming again recently and strained the underarm muscle on the operated side; naturally I thought the pain and lumpiness were due to recurrent cancer. I worry my long-suffering husband when I suspect I have detected secondary growths, and I am full of remorse when I find he is still worrying about something I've already forgotten.

I had a difficult time when I started writing this book. I'd put my cancer to the back of my mind and I was getting on with my life when the book brought it all to the fore again. The good part was that I found that the outlook for women with breast cancer was much more hopeful than I'd thought, and that the number of deaths from breast cancer was finally beginning to decrease. I made many new friends while visiting hospitals, self-help groups, cancer care centres, hospices, and the homes of women kind enough to allow me to come and discuss their breast cancer with them. I am very grateful to all those who spared the time to talk to me.

What this book is about

This book is not intended to be a medical textbook covering everything there is to know about breast cancer; nor can it answer every possible question a woman or a man with a breast lump may ask. It is for those who have little or no medical knowledge and who want to read something about the cancer they have or think they may have, and for their relatives and friends.

How to read this book

I am one of those people who have to read books from the beginning right through to the end. I can't just dip. On the assumption that you may be the same I have kept the least pleasant aspect of breast cancer (the possibility of secondary cancer) almost to the end in Chapter 14, *which you don't have to read.* What is right for some people is wrong for others. Some of us prefer to know the worst, even if it may never happen. Others of us prefer to put our heads in the sand. And why not? It is our choice. If you want to read this book straight through to the end that's fine. If you want to leave out Chapter 14, it is equally fine. As long as you get the message that there's hope, and that there are lots of us out there in exactly the same boat. We all have similar fears, whether we are doctors, teachers, housewives, journalists, actresses or whatever we are.

You may have a tough time reading some of the more medical chapters. There are lots of unfamiliar words to get to grips with if you want to understand what breast specialists are talking about (though the Glossary at the end of the book should help). Accounts of how breasts develop, what hormones do, and what cancer is, can be heavy going. You can skip those bits and come back to them later, if you find you want to read them after all.

The rest of the book

After this introduction there is a description of the normal breast and how it develops. This helps to explain why breasts are more vulnerable to things that cause cancer (carcinogens) at different stages. Benign (non-cancerous) breast problems are much more common than cancer, and an account of them follows. Chapters on the history, possible causes and diagnosis of breast cancer are followed by chapters on what to expect when you go to hospital, who's who, and descriptions of surgery, radiotherapy, chemotherapy and hormone treatment for breast cancer. A review of complementary therapies is followed by chapters on breast reconstruction, the psychological aspects of breast cancer, and the work situation. Chapter 14 covers recurrent and secondary cancer, and Chapter 15 concludes the book.

There are sections about male breast cancer in the appropriate chapters. In this country there are about 200 cases of male breast cancer each year, compared with nearly 30,000 cases in women. The number of male breast cancers has varied little in the last 20 years, while in women the rate of occurrence (the incidence) of breast cancer is still increasing (see Chapter 3). An account of the very much more frequent gynaecomastia (benign enlargement of the male breast) is found in Chapter 2.

Treatment under the NHS

In spite of all our grumbles we are very fortunate in the UK: we still receive treatment without the cost being a major consideration, as it is in the USA for example – though even here things are changing. If you have breast cancer you are treated almost as quickly in an NHS hospital as if you went privately, and your treatment is as good or better. Most NHS hospitals have the big advantage of having all the specialities under one roof, and treatment in the various departments can be easily co-ordinated. Some private patients find that no-one co-ordinates their treatment and they have to organise the liaison themselves.

However, as an NHS patient, you would probably have to wait a very long time for breast reconstruction, if you didn't have it carried out at the same time as your cancer was removed. It would be expensive to have breast reconstruction privately, but there wouldn't be the same long delay, nor would you have to face all the waiting in out-patient departments. If you have your own health insurance or sufficient funds, and have chosen to have your operation carried out privately, you can decide at any stage to change to treatment under the NHS.

Doctors – he or she?

I am a doctor, and this book is supportive of doctors. Of course we make mistakes, are often hurried and brusque, and sometimes insensitive. Breast cancer needs treatment by doctors, and it does women with breast cancer no good for the media to undermine the medical profession to the extent that women are afraid to seek treatment. Too often only the unfortunate minority who are *not* well treated are considered newsworthy, while little is written about the many women who are treated speedily and sympathetically. The UK has among the highest death rate from breast cancer in the world (see Chapter 3). Until recently about a third of British women did not seek medical advice until their cancer was advanced, compared with about 10% in Scandinavia and the USA. This must have made a major contribution to our high number of deaths from breast cancer – the likelihood of survival is less when the cancer is advanced before treatment starts. Although some breast cancers are missed by GPs, particularly in younger women in whom they are uncommon (see Chapter 3), most women with breast lumps are referred to a specialist without delay.

About 50% of medical students in the UK are female, but all too few of them make it to the top to become consultants. Most of the specialists are therefore men (though there are more women specialists in certain departments like radiotherapy); I have therefore chosen to use 'he' to refer to doctors throughout this book, rather than the inelegant 'they' or 'he or she'. I apologise to anyone who feels strongly about this. It is up to all of us to push for more women in top medical appointments, as well as in other professions.

1

The normal adult breast and its development

The adult breast

Adult female breasts extend further than you might think. They lie on the pectoral muscles of the chest and stretch from the second rib, which at the front is just below the collar bone, down to the sixth rib. In front they stretch from the edge of the breast bone to the midline under the armpit. They have a triangular extension into the armpit (axilla), known as the axillary tail (see Figure 1).

In most women the nipple sticks up above the skin and is capable of erection when excited, cold or irritated. It is surrounded by the areola, the circle of skin whose exact colour and amount of surrounding hair varies from woman to woman. The little knobs on the areola, Montgomery's tubercles, are glands that moisten the nipple during suckling.

Much of the breast consists of fat which is held in place by Cooper's ligaments – sheets of strong, fibrous tissue. These loosen with age, hence the sagging breasts of older women. The milk-producing breast tissue is composed of 12–20 lobules (see Figure 2, p. 6).

Milk passes along ducts (fine tubes) which lead into the wider lactiferous sinuses; these open in several places on the nipple. A tiny

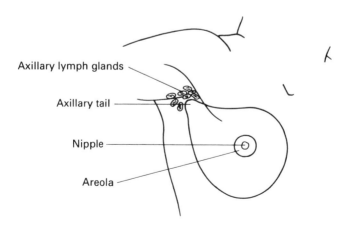

Figure 1 The female breast

amount of milky fluid, too little to be noticed, is secreted during adult life. If ducts become blocked for any reason, the secretions cannot get out; the ducts then enlarge forming cavities called cysts (see Chapter 2). The ducts together with their lobules are called TDLUs (terminal duct lobular units). It is from these that breast cancers develop (Chapter 4).

Breast development

In both boys and girls the breasts start to develop during the seventh week of pregnancy. The major ducts, which are formed between 13 and 20 weeks, end in small sacs, but milk-producing lobules do not start to form until puberty. Hormones in the mother's blood cross the placenta, and in some babies the levels are so high that for a short time after birth their breasts enlarge and produce so-called 'Witch's Milk'. After birth the mother's hormones are no longer available, so the baby's breasts return to an inactive state until puberty.

In girls of about ten years of age, the tissue under the nipple begins to grow forming a rounded breast bud, and the areola darkens. In some girls the blood vessels enlarge so much in order to bring more blood to the developing breast that one breast or both may appear blue for a time. This stage of breast development is complete when a girl reaches about 15, but the lobules do not finally mature until the end of the first pregnancy.

Boys develop a little breast tissue which has breast ducts but no lobules. Breast enlargement (gynaecomastia) is normal during the hormonal changes of puberty, when it often occurs on one side at a time. It usually goes away without treatment, but occasionally, if it persists, an operation maybe requested to remove the excess tissue, especially if it is one-sided.

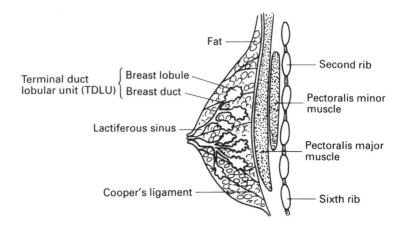

Figure 2 Cross-section of breast

However we try to come to terms with breast cancer and minimise the psychological effects of mastectomy or lumpectomy, it is difficult to get away from the fact that we distinguish between boys and girls, men and women, in jeans and loose T-shirts by looking to see whether or not they have breasts. Of course there are other differences – but it is the presence of breasts that confirms our sex to the onlooker.

Abnormalities of development

Breast development is often asymmetrical (lop-sided) and one breast may develop before the other. Many women have one breast slightly larger than the other; some have as much as two bra sizes difference between the two sides. Sometimes, instead of the nipple standing up from the breast, it is inverted (pulled in). This is common in children before puberty and in men, but in most girls the nipple becomes everted (turned out) as the breast develops. If you have always had one or both nipples inverted, this is normal for you and is nothing to worry about. However, you should go to see your doctor if your previously everted nipple becomes drawn in. A change like this could be a sign of underlying cancer (see Chapter 6 on diagnosis) – though there are other non-cancerous causes.

Both men and women may have an accessory (extra) nipple, and sometimes an extra breast may be present. These may occur in the armpit, but can be anywhere on the 'milk line', an imaginary line stretching from the armpit, through the position of the normal breasts, over the abdomen to the groin. (This is the line along which the multiple mammary glands of animals like dogs and cats develop.) Extra nipples or breasts can be removed if you think they are unsightly, or if an extra breast becomes swollen and uncomfortable during pregnancy. Rarely one or both breasts do not develop.

Hormones

Hormones are essential for the development of our breasts; they also play an important role in the development of breast cancer and in its treatment (see Chapters 4 and 8). It is useful therefore to know something about them.

Hormones are chemical substances mainly produced in our endocrine glands. These include the thyroid gland which produces thyroxin, the pancreas which produces insulin, and the ovaries which produce the female sex hormones, oestrogen and progesterone. Hormones are usually stored in the glands and released into the blood stream as the body requires them. The pituitary gland, a pea-sized gland at the base of the brain, controls many of these glands and has been referred to as 'the leader of the endocrine orchestra'. It is controlled in turn by a part of the brain called the hypothalamus – 'the conductor of the endocrine orchestra'.

Female sex hormones

Oestrogen and progesterone are responsible for the changes of puberty including breast development, and for menstruation and the features of pregnancy. Oestrogen is produced in the ovary during the whole of the menstrual cycle, and in the second half of the cycle progesterone is produced as well.

Hormones often have effects other than the obvious ones. Male and female sex hormones, for example, influence the development of our brains, and oestrogen is important for maintaining bone structure. The lack of female hormones after the menopause is one of the reasons for the osteoporosis (bone thinning) which makes older women more liable to fractures.

Women also produce some male hormones (androgens) in their adrenal glands. These can be converted to oestrogen in other tissues, particularly fat, under the influence of enzymes (substances which help chemical reactions) called aromatases.

Oestrogen in excess of the body's requirements is released into the blood stream and is broken down in the liver to an inactive form. Liver damage, for example due to alcoholism, results in high oestrogen levels and is thought to be the reason that alcohol increases the risk of breast cancer (see Chapter 5). High oestrogen levels due to liver failure are one cause of male breast enlargement (see Chapter 2).

Oestrogen receptors (ER)

Not all cells are affected by each hormone. Only those that have special molecules called receptors, either on their surface or inside them, will respond. Breast cells have receptors for several hormones, the most important of which are oestrogen and progesterone.

Oestrogen receptors (shortened to ER because oestrogen is spelt *estrogen* in the USA where the term was coined) are of great significance in breast cancer. Removing all sources of oestrogen or giving an anti-oestrogen like Tamoxifen to women whose cancers have high ER levels and need oestrogen for their continued growth can stop them growing, or even make them go away altogether.

Sex hormones and development of the lobules

Oestrogen is necessary for full development of the ducts but only for the first stages of development of the lobules. Progesterone is required for their completion. The first menstrual cycles are anovulatory – this means that they do not result in the production of ova (eggs) – and progesterone is not secreted. Once ovulatory cycles occur, progesterone is secreted and more mature lobules form in the breast.

Other hormones play a more minor role in breast development. They include insulin from the pancreas, growth hormone and prolactin from the pituitary gland, and steroids from the adrenal glands.

Although overproduction or failure to break down any of these hormones may influence the development of breast cancer, oestrogen is by far the most important.

Menstruation and pregnancy

Breasts undergo changes with each menstrual period. Some women's breasts become so tense and painful they require treatment (see Chapter 2), while others barely notice any difference.

During pregnancy the breast approximately doubles in weight, and development of the lobules is completed during this time. By the last three months of pregnancy, the lobules are developed fully and start to secrete a small amount of milk, not usually noticeable to the mother. Until the end of the first pregnancy, the lobules are therefore still immature, and immature tissues are more susceptible to cancer-promoting influences. The sooner the first pregnancy comes after the onset of menstruation (menarche), the shorter the time immature breasts are exposed to carcinogens.

During breast-feeding the lobules swell up with milk-producing cells. Once the baby is weaned, the breasts gradually return to their resting state, though a few cells can be seen to contain milk proteins under the microscope months or years later.

Involution

The term 'involution' covers both the return to normal after the end of breast feeding, and the gradual replacement of breast tissue by fat which starts at about the age of 35. The dense breast tissue of young women does not lend itself as well to mammography (see Chapter 6) and tiny cancers are difficult to detect in their breasts by this method. This is the reason that mammography is not offered under the NHS until a woman is 50, by which time the breast consists largely of fat. If a lump is found in the breast of a young woman she is more likely to be referred for ultrasound (see Chapter 6).

The blood and lymphatic systems

All the organs of the body are supplied with oxygen, sugar and other nutrients by way of blood flowing through the arteries. When the body has used the oxygen, the blood returns in the veins to the lungs to be re-oxygenated. Most fluid in the tissues is absorbed by capillaries (the smallest blood vessels) and thence passes into the veins.

A further system exists to return the remaining fluid to the circulating blood. This is the lymphatic system. It consists of thin walled lymphatics (tubes) all over the body which return the lymphatic fluid (lymph) to a vein in the neck via the thoracic duct (a large lymphatic in the chest).

Lymph glands (nodes)

Small, bean-shaped structures called lymph glands or nodes are scattered in groups along the course of the lymphatic vessels. These are very important parts of our immune system. Debris, bacteria and dead cells in the tissues are taken up by certain cells (macrophages) and brought to the lymph glands for destruction.

Immune protection against cancer

Lymph glands also contain plasma cells (which produce antibodies against a variety of diseases) and T-lymphocytes, cells that are vital for combating certain infections. The AIDS virus attacks these cells so that patients with AIDS are very prone to infections which would not affect a normal healthy adult. T-lymphocytes are also responsible for recognizing foreign cells, and are thus involved in the rejection of kidney and bone marrow grafts, if the tissue is not sufficiently like the patient's own.

T-lymphocytes also recognize and destroy our own cells when they become abnormal. NK cells (Natural Killer cells) are large lymphocytes with a similar function. A few of our normal cells become malignant under the influence of all the things that may cause cancer, like environmental radiation and smoking. Our immune system is geared to recognise that these are no longer normal cells. T-lymphocytes, together with NK cells and other substances produced by the body, stop them developing into tumours and kill them. One of the ways to avoid cancer may be to increase the efficiency of our immune systems by adopting a healthier life-style.

The principal group of glands in the lymphatic drainage of the breast is in the armpit (see Figure 1, p. 5). Other lymphatics drain towards the glands near the breast bone or those above the collar bone. Unfortunately cancer cells can travel along lymphatics with the lymph. They can then form secondary tumours in the lymph glands, or spread elsewhere in the body. If you have a breast lump, the doctor will feel under your arms to see whether there are enlarged glands due to cancer having spread there. However, lymph glands in your armpit may swell up for other reasons – for example due to glandular fever or an infected cut in the hand.

2

Benign breast conditions

If you find a lump in your breast and you are wondering if it could be cancer, take heart. In nine out of ten cases it won't be – though you may still need an operation to remove it. There are several causes of lumps in the breast other than cancer. By far the commonest is fibrocystic change or benign breast disease.

Fibrocystic change

Fibrocystic change involves scarring (fibrosis), the formation of cavities containing fluid (cysts), and an increase in the number of cells (hyperplasia). This type of change can be found in the breasts of at least 60% of women, so it is regarded by many as a non-disease, and part of the normal ageing process. It is therefore called by some doctors ANDI – Aberrations of Normal Development and Involution.

The cause of fibrocystic change is uncertain, though it is thought to be due to hormonal changes. Under the microscope it is seen to involve the whole breast, and it makes some women's breasts feel lumpy all over; however, sometimes only one firm area can be felt. This is not a tumour (see Chapter 4); it may be an area of fibrosis and hyperplasia with tiny cysts, or it may be one large cyst. The doctor will probably want to draw off some cells to be sure it is benign, using a fine needle attached to a hypodermic syringe. This is called a fine needle aspirate (FNA) (see Chapter 6). If the result is not conclusive, it may be necessary to remove part of the lump (a biopsy; see Chapter 6), or all of it, and examine it under the microscope to make sure no cancer is present.

Breast cysts

Single, large cysts are commonest in the ten years before the menopause, though they may also occur in younger women. If the lump turns out to be a cyst, it may only be necessary to draw off the fluid using a fine needle. Sometimes the cyst refills once or twice and has to be drained again, and further cysts may develop in the same or the other breast. If it keeps on refilling the cyst needs to be removed. If the fluid contains blood, it will be examined to be sure it does not contain cancer cells – though cancers in cysts are uncommon.

Some years before I actually had cancer, I found a lump in my left breast while having a shower after work. I was sure it was cancer and felt in my armpit on that side to see if it had already spread to my lymph glands. I telephoned one of my surgical colleagues and arranged to see him the next morning. Neither my husband nor I slept that night. When my colleague told me he thought the lump was a cyst, almost certainly benign, and that he needed to insert a needle to draw off the fluid, I was terrified I would make a fool of myself – calling out or even fainting. To my surprise, it was no more painful than having blood taken. I felt where the cyst had been while he was labelling the specimen of murky-looking fluid to be sent to the laboratory. The lump had gone completely, and it did not recur. I'd been afraid to hope the surgeon was right, but the cytologist (see Chapter 7) reported that the cyst was benign, as are practically all breast cysts.

New cysts usually stop appearing after the menopause, but the breasts of women on hormone replacement therapy (HRT) remain active, so they may develop further cysts. Always see your doctor if you develop a new lump. You need to be sure the new one is a cyst and not a cancer which should be removed while it is still small.

Cysts can come and go, filling up so you feel them and then disappearing by the time you see the specialist. Don't worry. He knows that cysts behave like that. He won't consider it a waste of time and would much rather you came and required no treatment other than reassurance, than risked missing a cancer.

Cysts do not develop into cancers, though single large ones are slightly more common in the breasts of women with cancer.

Atypical changes

Sometimes when a breast lump, which has been removed for fibrocystic change, is examined under the microscope, the cells are seen to be disorderly instead of arranged in neat rows, and all shapes and sizes instead of being more or less uniform. This is called 'atypia', and it is not yet cancer, though its presence increases the risk of cancer developing later (see Chapter 5). The specialist will therefore arrange to continue to see such patients regularly, rather than discharging them when their wound has healed.

Benign breast tumours

In Chapter 4, the difference between benign and malignant tumours (cancers) is explained, but essentially a benign breast tumour needs only to be removed, and neither radiotherapy nor chemotherapy are required. If it is removed completely it will not recur at the same site, nor will it spread elsewhere in the body. Cancer is very uncommon under the age of 25, but benign tumours are not at all unusual in young women and girls.

There are several types of benign breast tumour, none of which are in any way dangerous.

Fibroadenomas

The commonest benign tumour is a fibroadenoma, sometimes called a 'breast mouse', because it seems to slip around in the breast as you feel it. The diagnosis can be made by drawing off some cells with a needle. In some specialist breast clinics, a cytologist is on hand to look at the cells immediately; otherwise you may have to wait a few days for the result. Many surgeons now consider that in a young woman it is quite safe to leave a fibroadenoma, unless she wants it removed. In women over 40 fibroadenomas are better taken out, since the incidence of cancer is higher at that age and it is best to be certain that the lump is quite benign.

Other types

Other types of benign tumour occur in the breast such as tumours of fat cells (called lipomas), and sebaceous cysts. These are lumps in the skin containing keratin, the material from which nails, hair and the outer covering of the skin are made. They can be removed if they are unsightly, but they have no medical importance.

Nipple discharge

Most causes of nipple discharge are benign, but you should see a doctor about it to be sure, especially if the discharge contains blood. Thick or greenish discharges may be unpleasant, but they are not serious.

Duct ectasia

In duct ectasia a breast duct becomes enlarged and there is inflammation around it. It may cause a swelling near the nipple, or it may produce a thick discharge. If treatment is required, the affected duct is removed in a small operation.

Milk-flow in the non-pregnant breast (galactorrhoea)

Some women who are not pregnant have a tiny amount of milk-flow from one or both nipples, with no known cause. All they need is reassurance that it is nothing serious. If it becomes an embarrassment, the large ducts under the nipple can be cut on the affected side, leaving a small scar. Breast feeding will not then be possible on that side.

More rarely the breasts of either men or women secrete milk because the pituitary gland is secreting large amounts of the hormone prolactin. A blood test can show whether this is the cause. It can usually be treated with the drug bromocriptine.

Duct papillomas

A duct papilloma is something like a wart. It develops inside one of the breast ducts and may cause bleeding or discharge from the nipple. Duct papillomas need to be removed in a small operation to be sure that no cancer is present, which also causes bleeding from the nipple.

Painful breasts (mastalgia)

There are three main types of breast pain:

- pain which is clearly related to the menstrual cycle;
- pain which comes and goes but is not cyclical;
- pain due to a cause outside the breast, like a sore rib.

Pain is not commonly a symptom of cancer, and women who have breast pain are no more likely to get cancer than any other woman. Some cancers of the breast are tender to the touch, but the majority are not.

Most of us can put up with tender breasts just before a period, but some women have such painful breasts they can't bear to be touched or hugged. Reducing the amount of drinks containing caffeine – like coffee, tea or cola – has helped some women. If you suffer from breast pain, try wearing a comfortable bra with good support, and a soft bra at night.

Women may develop painful breasts when they change to an underwired bra which cuts into the breast, or when they take up a new, strenuous exercise, or put on weight so that their heavier breasts pull more on the supporting ligaments. A better bra can often help, or losing weight, if that is the cause.

Breast pain tends to disappear with the menopause, unless you are taking hormone replacement therapy (HRT) when the pain may continue. For women on the Pill it is worth trying another type, or changing to a different form of contraception.

Most women are able to put up with the discomfort once they are reassured they don't have cancer. For those for whom none of these simple measures work, there are drugs that may help.

Medical treatment of breast pain

The treatment with the fewest side-effects is Evening Primrose Oil. This is based on the finding that some women with severe breast pain have lower-than-normal levels of the fatty acids which are present in Evening

Primrose Oil. The tablets need to be taken for at least three months before you can be sure whether they are helping or not.

If this is not successful some hospitals have breast clinics specializing in the treatment of breast pain. Hormone treatments with Danazol, which interferes with the production of sex hormones, or bromocriptine, which decreases the secretion of the hormone prolactin, can be tried. They both may have unpleasant side-effects: growth of facial hair, weight gain or acne in the case of Danazol; nausea and dizziness in the case of bromocriptine. They are therefore given only in short courses, after which the pain may go away and not return.

Some GPs are not very sympathetic, and regard women complaining of breast pain as neurotic. Change to a GP who is more understanding.

Fat necrosis

Breasts stick out, and so they are liable to suffer mild injury. Sometimes a group of fat cells is so damaged that it dies. This is called 'fat necrosis'. A scar is formed which feels like a hard lump, and when the scar contracts, the overlying skin can pucker and be pulled down. Since puckering of the skin over a lump is a possible sign of cancer, areas of fat necrosis can be hard to distinguish from cancer until the lump is examined under the microscope. It is one of the pleasures in life for a pathologist (see Chapter 7) to be able to report that what was thought to be cancer is only an area of fat necrosis, and not malignant at all.

Other causes of breast lumps

Abscesses in the breast generally form red, tender areas rather than lumps. They occur most often in women who are breast-feeding, particularly if they have a cracked nipple. Abscesses in women who are not breast-feeding are more often associated with a lump, and may not be hot and tender. Infections like tuberculosis (TB) may be the cause of a breast lump, especially in those countries where TB is common.

The pathologist's report

The surgeon may be fairly confident that your lump is benign, but only after the pathologist has carefully examined all the tissue can they be sure that no cancer is present. Women go through a great deal of anguish before they first go to their doctor, and we all fear that any breast lump must be cancer. The few extra days you have to wait for the final all clear can be almost too much to bear. If you feel you have been waiting too long for the result, ask your GP to phone the hospital – or phone the clinic yourself.

Yet another lump

Benign breast lumps can recur at a different place in the same breast or in the other breast, and the new lump will probably also be benign. However, every lump should be taken seriously and you should go to the doctor as soon as you find one.

Breast enlargement in men

Gynaecomastia is breast enlargement in boys or men, and is common at puberty. It may occur in adult men without any detectable cause, while others have gynaecomastia due to the side-effects of certain medicines such as cimetidine (prescribed for stomach ulcers), or the use of substances such as marijuana or ginseng. A few have a more serious medical cause, such as a diseased liver which does not break down the small amounts of oestrogen men produce, so that they have high blood-levels of female sex hormones. Some have a tumour of the lung or testis which secretes hormones that cause breast enlargement.

Men can, of course, also develop breast cancer – though only about 200 a year do so in the whole of the UK. Most men are not aware of this, and are liable to ignore a breast lump until their cancer is advanced.

3

Breast cancer past and present

The history of breast cancer

Cancer of the breast is not a new disease. It was mentioned in Egyptian papyruses as far back as 3000 BC, in Indian writings of 2000 BC, and in those of Greek and Roman physicians in the fourth century BC. In the first century AD there were accounts of surgery for breast cancer by Celsius, a Roman living in what is now Provence.

The great physician Hippocrates, who was born on the Greek island of Kos in 460 BC, proposed that we are composed of four humours. Each humour was associated with an element – blood with air, yellow bile with fire, black bile with earth, and phlegm with water. He and Galen, a Greek physician born in Asia Minor in 130 AD, dominated medical thought for centuries. They taught that cancer was a disease of the whole body caused by bad humours, particularly black bile. Galen claimed to have had success by treating the excess of black bile medically, and both of them thought that surgery was of little value. Surgery was also discouraged by the Church which claimed miraculous cures in women spending the night in a church.

In medieval times various unpleasant remedies were used. These included purging (cleaning out the bowel with enemas or laxatives) and bleeding. Some involved application of herbs, ointments, the urine of a young maiden, or oil of frogs made by baking them with butter in their mouths. Laying on of hands by royalty was also recommended. It was recognised that breast cancer most often occurred in postmenopausal women; it was therefore considered to be due to stopping the release of menstrual 'poisons'. Indeed, it was thought that menstrual 'effluvium' disposed of an excess of black bile, and there were many suggested ways of restarting menstruation.

In the seventeenth century an account of a housemaid 'catching' cancer from her employer was published and regarded as positive proof of its infectious nature. Right up to the eighteenth century patients with breast cancer were not admitted to public hospitals because of the mistaken idea it could be passed from person to person in that way.

Surgery for breast cancer was, however, still performed, usually preceded by 'cleansing' – purging and bleeding, two activities likely to weaken the patient. In the sixteenth century removal of the whole breast, together with the underlying chest muscle, was advocated. Later on, removal of the lymph glands in the armpit was also advised. At a time when anaesthesia was unknown, mastectomy was a horrendous procedure. However, some skilled surgeons could remove a breast within two minutes.

When lymphatics were discovered in the seventeenth century, breast cancer was thought to arise within them. That cancer did not arise within lymphatics but was spread by them was recognised in the eighteenth century. Surgeons therefore thought that they could cure breast cancer by removing the breast, the chest muscles and the lymph nodes in the armpit. Anaesthesia was introduced in 1846 and this operation, now called radical mastectomy, was popularised by the American surgeon Halstead, towards the end of the last century. In defence of those who advocated radical mastectomy, it must be remembered that women would have been embarrassed at seeing a doctor on so delicate a matter; surgery was still a formidable undertaking before antiseptics and antibiotics. Many would have waited to seek advice until their cancer was far advanced, and had invaded the underlying muscle or burst through the skin.

By the end of the nineteenth century it was known that cancer could spread in the blood stream as well as by lymphatics. It was recognised that this might occur very early and that tiny outposts of cancer could exist elsewhere in the body. The concept of the 'seed and soil' was developed – that though cancer cells may spread, conditions had to be right for them to take hold and grow into secondary tumours. None the less, radical mastectomies continued to be performed. Some surgeons carried out even more extensive procedures. These 'supra-radical' mastectomies included removing the collar bone to take away the lymph glands sheltering behind it, and removing portions of the ribs to take away the lymph nodes running along the side of the breast bone.

X-rays were discovered by Roentgen in 1875 and radiotherapy was used within a year to treat breast cancer. In the late 1920s, Keynes in the UK published his findings on treating breast cancer by irradiation alone. In France, Baclesse and his colleagues used lumpectomy followed by radiotherapy from the late 1930s, and then radiotherapy alone. In the 1940s McWhirter advocated simple mastectomy (removal of the breast without the underlying muscles) followed by radiotherapy. Many doctors still thought that anything other than radical mastectomy was little short of heresy, but, the operation of lumpectomy and removal of the lymph glands in the armpit (axillary clearance) gained ground as more and more women refused mastectomy.

In the 1980s, large studies showed that women who had a lumpectomy were as likely to survive as women who had a mastectomy – although the chance of having a local recurrence in the breast was increased. Some women therefore needed a mastectomy later, but their survival was not affected. Now that it is usual to follow lumpectomy by radiotherapy, local recurrence is less common.

Hormone treatment was ushered in by the Scottish surgeon Beatson at the end of the nineteenth century. He showed that when the ovaries of some breast-cancer patients were removed, their tumours got smaller. In the 1950s, removal of the adrenal glands (which produce sex hormones that can be converted into oestrogen), or of the pituitary gland (which controls production of sex hormones by the ovaries) was introduced.

In the 1960s the American physician, Jensen, showed that in order to respond to hormones, normal cells and cancer cells have to possess molecules on to which the hormones can latch. In the case of breast cancer, these are oestrogen receptors (ER). A cancer with high levels of oestrogen receptors requires oestrogen for its continued growth. If all sources are removed, or the patient is given an anti-oestrogen like Tamoxifen, the tumour stops growing, may get smaller or even disappear altogether, and secondary cancers do not form. Some breast cancers also have high levels of receptors for the sex hormone, progesterone. They are important for the production of oestrogen receptors.

Breast cancer: the statistics

Breast cancer is a disease which occurs mainly in Western, developed countries. Each year over half a million women develop breast cancer worldwide, with 50% of these cases occurring in North America and Europe, which contain less than 20% of the total female population.

In the UK, breast cancer is the most common female cancer. There are about 105,000 women who have it, or who have been operated on for it, at any one time (its prevalence). The number of new cases of breast cancer in women in England and Wales (the incidence) was 28,812 in 1990 (the most recent year for which accurate figures are available), with 13,634 deaths. In comparison, there were 4,310 cancers of the cervix, with 1,781 deaths. In the same year, there were 198 cases of male breast cancer with 107 deaths. In the UK women have a lifetime risk of breast cancer of 1 in 12. In the USA the risk is higher (1 in 9). In both countries the number of cases is rising year by year, as shown in Figure 3, p. 20.

This can partly be explained by the fact that women are living longer so that there are more of us. In addition, if the population ages there will be more cases because older women are more likely to get breast cancer – as well as other common cancers.

Almost 80% of breast cancers occur in women over 50. At the turn of the century the expectation of life for women was just under 50, compared

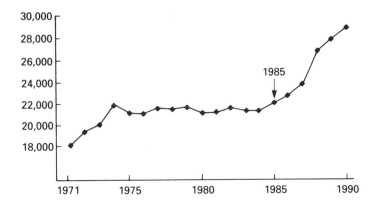

Figure 3 New cases of breast cancer in England and Wales 1971–90

with 82 today. In those days most women wouldn't have lived long enough to have developed cancer. Now that there is a three-yearly NHS mammography service, tiny cancers which might never have grown large enough to require treatment are being diagnosed. This may produce an apparent increase in breast cancer rates in screened women. As the years go by, this will even itself out, and fewer advanced cancers will be detected. However, the recent sharp increase in new cases started in 1985, before screening under the NHS was introduced in 1991.

There is a regional variation in breast cancer incidence in post-menopausal women in the UK, with more cases in the wealthier south. One explanation is that as women get richer they tend to have their first baby later, as well as having a diet containing more animal fats, both possible risk factors for breast cancer (see Chapter 5). This pattern is not seen in younger, premenopausal women.

Five-year survival figures are always quoted as an achievable time to follow up what has happened to patients, given the mobility of modern populations. The five-year survival of all women with breast cancer in the UK is 62%; the figures are better for small cancers which have not spread and worse for advanced cancers (see Chapter 4).

In 1990, the UK had the highest number of deaths from breast cancer worldwide, with a mortality rate of 28.33 per 100,000 population. In Europe, Denmark was very close behind with 28.11 per 100,000, then Ireland with 26.86 and Belgium with 26.83. These figures can be compared with a mortality of 19.44 per 100,000 in France, 15.35 in Spain and 15.33 in Greece. Japan, also a highly developed country, had a breast cancer mortality of 5.8 per 100,000 – a figure only one fifth of ours.

In Europe, the occurrence rate of new cases of breast cancer (the incidence) was highest in Switzerland, with 72.2 cases per 100,000 population, 62.4 in France, 59.7 in Southern Ireland, 59.6 in Italy and 54.0 in England and Wales. The highest rate worldwide was in Hawaii with 93.9 per 100,000, followed by 77.5 per 100,000 in the USA. The lowest incidence was among non-Jews in Israel with 14.0 per 100,000, then Kuwait with 15.9, China 19.1 and Japan 22.0.

While Japanese women in Japan have an incidence of 22.0 per 100,000, when they emigrate to the USA the figure rises to 36.2. In the UK, ethnic groups compose about 6% of the population, and – as in the USA – immigrants are beginning to have the same cancer incidence and mortality as the white resident population. In India the incidence of breast cancer is low, (24.1 per 100,000), less than half that of the UK, with a correspondingly low mortality. Figures on the occurrence of breast cancer in ethnic minority groups in the UK are not yet available, but their mortality from breast cancer is now 70–80% of that of the local population, and seems to be increasing in younger women. Factors other than the country of residence are important: Jews born in Israel, for example, have incidence rates higher than those in Europe (76.7 per 100,000), while their non-Jewish neighbours have the lowest incidence in the world.

Why is mortality so high in the UK?

The reasons for the high mortality rate in the UK are not clear. The incidence here is much lower than in the USA, but mortality is higher. Women with breast cancer in this country are more likely to put off going to the doctor and there is less health awareness. In Norway, only 9% of women have advanced cancers when they are first seen. In the USA the figure is 11%. There, most women have private health insurance and it can be a condition of continuing cover that they have regular health check-ups. In the UK, up to 35% of women may have advanced cancer (which has a lower survival rate; see Chapter 4) when they first go to the doctor. This may be because they delay before seeking advice; it may also be that a combination of genetic and environmental factors causes us to develop more aggressive tumours, more likely to have grown large before we notice them, more likely to kill us.

Breast cancer mortality in England and Wales has been falling since 1989 – from 14,008 in 1989 to 12,830 in 1994 – having been rising steadily before that, as shown in Figure 4, p. 22. The actual fall is probably greater still, because mortality from breast cancer in women over 70 is still increasing, and this masks the improvement in survival of younger women. Depending on the year in question and the way the figures are calculated, Denmark seems to have the second highest mortality in

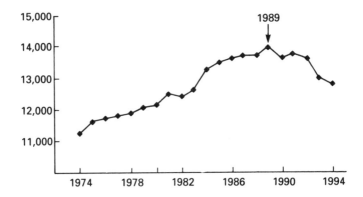

Figure 4 Breast cancer mortality in England and Wales 1974–94

Europe, with Holland and Belgium close behind. It seems most unlikely that the main reason for the high mortality in our four countries is that we have worse medical treatment than elsewhere.

Though breast cancer is the most common cause of death in women aged 35–44 (with 698 deaths in England and Wales in 1994), there were also 585 deaths from heart disease. In this age-group mortality from breast cancer has fallen since 1988, although the annual rate of occurrence is still rising, though not more than in other age groups. Increased breast awareness, and improvement in diagnosis and treatment, will be major contributory factors to further improvement in survival.

Breast cancer in perspective

The female population in England and Wales is just over 26 million. If we look at the major causes of death in women, we see that in 1994 there were 126,182 female deaths from diseases of the circulatory system – mainly heart attacks and strokes. In comparison, there were 12,830 deaths from breast cancer (nearly 1200 fewer than in 1989), and 11,009 deaths from lung cancer. When we come to think about what we should do to prevent breast cancer we should also think about reducing the large number of deaths from heart disease and lung cancer. When assessing risks, we often comment on the danger of crossing the road. In 1993 (1994 figures are not yet available) there were 864 deaths in women from road traffic accidents – not in the same league as heart disease, breast or lung cancer.

Why are the figures out of date?

It is easier to collect figures on *mortality* from death certificates, so information on mortality is published by the Office of Population, Censuses and Surveys (OPCS) only one to two years in arrears. In the UK we expect a slight hiccup in figures over the next few years while changes in the way deaths are computerised work their way through the system. Trends will therefore be more difficult to assess.

Figures on cancer *incidence* are published four to five years in arrears. This is because all new cancers are reported to regional cancer registries. National figures are not published by the OPCS until all of the cancer registries in the country have sent in their figures, and it takes some time to collate and check the data from all these centres.

Doubt and certainty

Friends often ask me why doctors can't seem to agree about breast cancer, why they don't speak with one voice. Why don't they make up their minds so that we could know where we stand? Why are articles in popular magazines and newspapers so certain, yet your book is so full of 'it may be' and 'it is possible that'? Wouldn't it be simpler if all doctors agreed on the correct treatment of breast cancer, and if everything in books and articles recommended the same operations and the same follow-up treatment?

As in so many fields, not only do experts not always agree, but opinions change in the light of new information and new research. There was a time when the standard treatment of breast cancer was radical mastectomy, with some surgeons recommending even more extensive surgery. Supra-radical mastectomy was based on the incorrect idea that breast cancer spread outwards from the tumour, so if you removed enough tissue you would eradicate all the tumour. Studies have now shown that women do not live any longer if they have mastectomy rather than lumpectomy, so many more are now offered less extensive surgery.

Breast reconstruction after cancer used to be frowned upon. Now it is often carried out, although the methods used are still subject to debate (see Chapter 10).

There is no easy answer to the question of how a woman with little medical knowledge should choose to have mastectomy or lumpectomy, or whether or not to have breast reconstruction. Some doctors recommend that the patient should assess the situation for herself, but it is not easy. I am an expert in one aspect of cancer – yet, to write this book, I had to read a vast amount to find out what is thought in the medical profession. Women are advised not to make up their minds at once; to think it over and talk to anyone they think might help.

Like many women, when it was confirmed I had cancer I just wanted it out of me as soon as possible. My cancer was small, and the surgeon recommended lumpectomy – but if he had suggested mastectomy instead, I am sure I would have agreed just to get it over and done with as soon as possible, and then regretted it later.

Stories and statistics

Stories, or anecdotal evidence, are reports of a few incidences of something happening which has not been scientifically investigated and which could have occurred by chance. For example, if you toss a coin thousands of times, it will fall 50% of the times on its head and 50% on its tail. If you toss it only five times, the coin could land four times on its head, by chance – and from this very limited 'experiment', your story, or anecdotal evidence, would (incorrectly) be that coins land on their heads 80% of the time.

Statisticians can put a value on the likelihood of a result being due to chance. The larger the number of tests carried out, the less likely it is that the results are due to chance. In order to be sure that changing our diet, giving up smoking or using a new treatment really prevents cancer or cures it, we must study a large number of people. If the likelihood of a treatment being successful entirely due to chance is less than about 1 in 20 it is said to be statistically significant.

If there are only a few cases, or it is just an impression or a gut feeling, the conclusion may be correct, but before applying it widely it needs to be tested further. At this stage the evidence is 'anecdotal', a series of cases not yet subjected to stringent testing. For doctors to feel confident in the results, trials are often carried out simultaneously in several hospitals or even several countries, so that there are enough patients in the study.

Retrospective and prospective studies

A *retrospective* study is one that is carried out using the case notes or memories of patients. For example, we could look at all women with breast cancer and read their notes to see at what age they had their first baby and compare them with a group of healthy women or a group of women who have come to hospital for a completely different disease and who do not have cancer. The advantage of using hospital notes is that you can go back many years and collect a large group of patients. The down side is that they may contain errors and sometimes get lost.

It is easier to avoid these problems in a *prospective* study. Here a group of people is followed up for a number of years to see which of them develops the disease being studied. Any factors which seem relevant, like diet and alcohol intake, are recorded. The advantage of this is that the people taking part in the study do not have to rely on their memory. The disadvantage is that it may take many years to get an answer. There is currently a study planned in several countries on women who are at high risk of getting breast cancer, those with close relatives who have developed breast cancer before the menopause. They will be given the anti-oestrogen Tamoxifen (see Chapter 9), to see whether it will reduce the number of breast cancers in this group. Other studies are investigating the length of time postmenopausal women should take Tamoxifen. It will be several years before enough results are available to assess the benefits and possible side-effects from long-term use of the drug, particularly in healthy but high risk, premenopausal women.

Placebo effect

We often feel better when a doctor takes over our care, even before he has done anything. Pills may seem to improve our symptoms before they could possibly have had time to take effect. This is called the 'placebo' effect (from the Latin *placere* to please). Harmless pills containing chalk or sugar (placebos) are sometimes made up and given to patients taking part in scientific tests, or 'controlled trials'. Numerous experiments have shown that some of the people who have the chalk pill or sugar tablet will get better. This may be by chance, since most diseases have their ups and downs, or an example of mind over matter. Whatever the reason, it is only when there is a statistically significant difference between the number of people getting better on the medicine and those getting better on the placebo that the treatment will be adopted for general use.

For some, 'placebo' is almost a dirty word. They suggest that it may be a bad thing for us to get better just because we *think* the treatment is doing us good. But that is what faith in our doctors is all about, and the placebo effect is a desirable part of the human condition. Haven't you ever felt your headache and tiredness vanish the minute a friend rings and says there's a party?

It is important, though, to distinguish between the effect of the medicine and the placebo effect. All drugs have some side-effects and there is no point in having a treatment which is no better than a sugar pill – or a few words of reassurance.

Controlled trials

We are influenced by how we *think* we should feel. We might either exaggerate the benefits or play down any unpleasant side-effects if we thought we were getting the newest treatment. Similarly, the doctor carrying out the trial might be prejudiced by his belief that the new treatment was better. To avoid bias, the patients who are to have the new treatment are selected not by the doctor but at random. This can be done by pulling numbers out of a hat, by taking alternate patients coming to the clinic, or by using a random numbers table to decide which patients have the treatment.

A controlled trial is where one group of patients has the treatment and one does not, or one has a new, improved treatment and the other group has the accepted one. The patients having the placebo or the old treatment act as a control for the patients having the new treatment. In a blind trial the patient does not know whether he or she is having the treatment or the placebo, or the old or new treatment, but the doctor does. A double blind trial is one in which neither the doctor nor the patient knows which group is having the new treatment. A blind trial is suitable for tests of tablets which can either be made to look alike or where neither the patients nor the doctors know which tablet is which. Where two forms of treatment, like surgery and chemotherapy, are compared everyone knows who is having which treatment; but which patient receives which treatment can be selected randomly.

It is a condition of all controlled trials that they must be passed by the hospital's ethical committee and that all patients must give their informed consent. This means that if you are invited to take part in a trial, you must be told what the trial is about, why it is being carried out, why you have been asked to take part and exactly how you will be involved. You can withdraw from a trial at any time if you change your mind. It should not affect the care your doctor will give you – though patients taking part in clinical trials tend to be seen more frequently, and problems are picked up sooner. Trials will be abandoned once it is absolutely clear that one of the treatments is superior.

Controlled trials and complementary medicine

In today's stressful society, there is undoubtedly a place for forms of treatment other than orthodox medicine. One of the criticisms orthodox doctors have of complementary medicine is that many complementary treatments have not been subjected to controlled trials. Of course, there are also many medicines in everyday use, such as aspirin for headache, which have never been tested in this way, but all new drugs and forms of treatment have to be subjected to controlled research.

Some complementary practitioners argue that it is immoral to deprive patients of treatment they know to work, and are unwilling to take part in such trials. However, there are numerous examples of people 'knowing' they were right. A century ago, everybody 'knew' that cupping, bleeding and purging were necessary for many different diseases. Surgeons 'knew' that the way to cure breast cancer was to carry out larger and larger operations, and they were unwilling to risk their patients' lives by carrying out a smaller operation. The less extensive operation of lumpectomy only became generally used when large, controlled trials showed that women who had lumpectomy survived just as long as those who had been treated by mastectomy.

Why don't they know?

Much is written in articles and books on breast cancer about the accompanying doubt and uncertainty. Many women are very angry that they are not given what they would regard as a straight answer and hard facts. Unfortunately, there is often no single correct answer, and the facts may be difficult to come by.

At a meeting of women determined to improve the facilities available for dealing with breast cancer, over and over I heard, '*Why* don't they know?' It was difficult to persuade them that you could contemplate your navel till the cows came home, and still not *know* which treatment was best. Doctors have to make a value-judgement about which new operation or new drug to try out, and then persuade women to take part in trials to find out which work best.

Even if you have no reservations about experiments on animals, in the end new treatments have to be tried out on humans. Until careful, controlled trials have been carried out no-one can predict the answer. We all have reservations about being guinea pigs for new methods of diagnosis and for new treatments, but how else can the answers be found?

It is understandable that women are angry that doctors are not infallible – but it is not reasonable.

My friends are always horrified when I say, 'Well, architects and lawyers make mistakes, heads of state and generals too'. They feel doctors should be perfect, but all doctors can do is their best in good faith. They can admit when they are wrong, and often that is what women want most of all, an honest admission of error. However, these days, when the next step is to the courts, everyone is always advised to say nothing, and patients may not have the satisfaction of a simple apology.

4

About breast cancer

What is cancer?

If you have never come into contact with someone who has had cancer, you may know very little about it – but you may have heard all sorts of old wives' tales. The name cancer comes from the Latin word for a crab, based on the way advanced breast cancer looked to the ancients, with enlarged blood vessels radiating out from it. It is also similar to a crab with claws of tumour growing into surrounding tissues.

A tumour is an abnormal growth of cells, and cancers are malignant tumours. This means that they can recur locally near the site from which they were removed, even if they seem to be removed completely, and they can spread elsewhere in the body.

- Cancers of the breast, skin, stomach, bowel, kidney, lungs and endocrine glands are called *carcinomas* (from the Greek *karkinos*, which also means a crab).
- Tumours of muscle and bone are called *sarcomas.*
- Cancers of blood-forming cells are called *leukaemias.*
- Tumours of lymph glands are called *lymphomas.*

Cancers of the breast do not interfere with any bodily functions, so until we find a lump we feel perfectly well. But, when breast cancers seed themselves elsewhere in the body – in the brain, lungs or liver – they can interfere with vital functions and become dangerous. However, not all cancers spread. Many malignant tumours, if they are detected and removed when they are small, do not recur and do not spread.

Growth control

The growth of normal cells in our body is very tightly controlled. We replace the worn-out cells of our skin, gut-lining and blood throughout our life, but once we reach adult size our liver, lungs and kidneys don't go on growing and growing. The body has a very complex system of growth-inducing factors and growth-suppressing factors which keep us approximately the same size – give or take a bit of fat. Only those parts of our bodies that are subjected to special needs continue to grow. Some organs, like the brain, never regrow when they are damaged; others, like the liver, will regrow a portion that is damaged or removed, as part of a surgical operation for example. Once the previous size is reached growth stops.

Growth during adulthood is called *hypertrophy*, when individual cells get larger – for example in the muscles of the uterus during pregnancy or in the legs of an athlete. At the end of pregnancy, or when an athlete stops exercising, the muscle cells return to their normal size. When tissues grow by making more cells, such as in the breast during pregnancy, this is called *hyperplasia.*

The growth control of cancers is defective. Even when their cells pile on top of each other and are squeezed into a small space, they continue to grow. However, cancers are not completely outside normal control: certain breast cancers, for example, ER-positive tumours (see Chapter 1), require oestrogen for their continued growth. They can therefore be treated either by removing the source of the oestrogen (the ovaries, for example), or by giving an anti-oestrogen drug like Tamoxifen.

Some cancers, like certain types in the thyroid gland, grow very slowly. Even if they have spread to form secondary tumours, they are compatible with a normal life span. In contrast, small-cell carcinomas of the lung grow and spread so fast it is not worthwhile removing the primary tumour. Even if only a small primary tumour is found, it is treated with chemotherapy (see Chapter 9) as if it had already spread. It is believed that breast cancers spread early in their course, so most women are treated with Tamoxifen or chemotherapy after surgery to prevent secondary tumours developing.

Benign and malignant tumours

Benign tumours are so called because on the whole they don't do you any harm. They don't invade the tissues around them and they don't spread. A fatty lump on your arm or abdomen may be unsightly but it doesn't affect your health. In some circumstances, however, benign tumours can cause trouble. A benign tumour situated in one of the chambers of the heart, for example, can obstruct the blood flow, and one in the brain can interfere with vital brain functions by raising the pressure inside the skull. Tumours in endocrine glands may overproduce their hormones and cause serious disease. A benign tumour can require emergency removal when it is in the intestine and causing a blockage.

Malignant tumours, cancers, can be dangerous in the same way as benign tumours – because of their position or overproduction of hormones – but in addition, they can invade surrounding tissues. They can seed themselves elsewhere in the body via the blood stream, the lymphatics and body cavities, and set up new satellite colonies of cancer cells. They are more difficult to remove completely, since tiny groups of cancerous cells can lurk in what looks to the surgeon like normal tissue. It is therefore necessary to remove a good margin of normal tissue to be sure any outlying cancer cells have been caught.

CIS (*Carcinoma in situ*)

Carcinoma *in situ* (CIS – from the Latin 'in the normal place') is a sort of half-way house, and it is sometimes called pre-cancer. In CIS, the cells in a breast TDLU (terminal duct lobular unit) are malignant, but they haven't yet broken out into the surrounding tissue (see Figure 5, p. 31). Areas of CIS are often undetectable to the touch but they can be picked up on mammograms (see Chapter 6), and specialists are seeing many more abnormalities of this type. CIS does not spread, does not form secondary tumours, and is not in some vital area like the brain and therefore cannot kill you; but in a high proportion of cases it will in time break through and become invasive. It is therefore potentially dangerous and needs to be removed. CIS is called either ductal carcinoma *in-situ* (DCIS) or lobular carcinoma *in-situ* (LCIS), depending on its appearance under the microscope.

CIS also occurs in other places in the body, such as on the cervix. In some countries, the detection of cervical CIS by regular cervical smears has reduced the number of invasive cancers of the cervix by up to 70%.

What causes breast cancer?

We don't know what causes breast cancer. We know quite a lot about the causes of other common cancers, such as lung and bowel cancer. It is established that smoking causes lung cancer, though occasionally it occurs in people who have never smoked nor been exposed to passive smoking. Cancer of the large bowel is common in the Western world where a highly refined, low-fibre diet is eaten, and is rare in developing countries where a high-fibre diet speeds up the passage of food down the bowel. This shortens exposure to bowel contents which are thought to contain natural carcinogens (substances that cause cancer). Some experts believe that a high-fibre diet also helps protect against breast cancer, because any carcinogens which may cause breast cancer are also hurried through the bowel, and don't stay long enough to get into the bloodstream.

Risk factors which may have a part to play in causing breast cancer are discussed in Chapter 5.

Prognosis

Prognosis is what is likely to happen to your disease. If your prognosis is very good you will live as long as if you didn't have cancer, and if it is bad you are unlikely to do so. Some types of cancer have an almost invariably

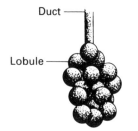

Duct

Lobule

In a normal duct the cells and nuclei are approximately the same size and shape

1. Normal breast duct and lobule

2. Normal breast duct cut in section

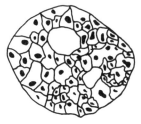

In CIS the ducts are swollen with irregular cells of all shapes and sizes but no cells have escaped into the surrounding tissues

3. Carcinoma *in situ* (CIS; ductal type)

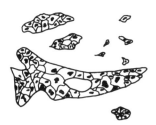

In invasive breast cancer streams of cancer cells invade the surrounding tissue. Some are making an attempt to form duct-like structures

4. Invasive breast cancer (ductal type)

Figure 5 The normal terminal duct breast lobular unit (TDLU), carcinoma *in situ* (CIS) and invasive breast cancer

good prognosis like many skin cancers and certain tumours of the thyroid. Breast cancer has the second-best prognosis of all specifically female cancers, with an average five-year survival of 62%.

How do doctors predict outcomes?

The most important features are:

- the size of the cancer;
- whether it has spread to the lymph nodes or elsewhere in the body;
- how closely it resembles normal breast tissue under the microscope.

31

Size

The smaller the tumour, the better the prognosis. Many cancers picked up by mammography (see Chapter 6) are too small to feel. These have an excellent prognosis. As a nation, we are very bad at seeking care early: too many women do not go to their doctor until their tumour is large. Once we are all used to having regular mammograms after the age of 50, this should help. In Scandinavia where 80–90% of women invited to have a mammogram attended, breast cancer mortality was reduced by 30–40%.

Spread (stage and node status)

With the removal of either the lump (lumpectomy) or the whole breast (mastectomy), some or all of the lymph glands in the armpit are also removed. Whether the tumour has spread to these glands is called the 'node status'. The fewer that contain cancer the better. Those with no tumour in their nodes have the best outlook. If the cancer has spread to fewer than four nodes, the outlook is still good; if more than four are involved, the outlook is worse. The future is less bright if the cancer has already spread to other parts of the body. Breast cancers, in which cancer cells are seen under the microscope in blood vessels and lymphatics, have a worse prognosis.

The extent of spread is called the stage of the cancer. CIS is sometimes called Stage 0.

- Stage 1: The cancer is confined to the breast;
- Stage 2: The axillary lymph nodes are involved;
- Stage 3: The cancer has spread into the overlying skin or underlying muscle;
- Stage 4: The cancer has spread elsewhere in the body.

Figures given for survival are only correct when large numbers of women are being considered. It is not possible to predict exactly how your cancer will behave, but looking at its stage gives an indication of whether you are likely to do well or badly. The overall five-year survival, combining all stages of breast cancer, is 62%. As you might expect, the prognosis for Stage 1 and Stage 2 cancers is better: 84% for Stage 1, and 71% for Stage 2. For patients with Stage 3 cancer (also called locally advanced cancer), the figure is 48%, and for Stage 4 disease it is 18%. No-one can tell whether someone will be among the 18% of Stage 4 patients who are going to survive at least five years, or among the 72% who are not.

The appearance of the cancer under the microscope (grade)

Grading is a system for seeing how closely the cancer resembles normal breast-tissue (in technical terminology, how well differentiated it is), and how fast it is growing. Under the microscope, malignant tumours may look very like normal tissue; these are called well differentiated. Other tumours are so unlike normal breast-tissue that it is hard to decide just what kind of cancer they are. They are called poorly differentiated if they are just recognisable, and undifferentiated if it is possible to say they are malignant but not identify their type. The number of cells which are dividing can be counted (this is called the mitotic index). Very malignant tumours are likely to have a lot of dividing cells if they are growing rapidly. The more primitive and undifferentiated the tumour looks under the microscope, the higher its grade is. High grade cancers are more likely to spread, and have a worse prognosis.

TNM classification

The UICC (Union Internationale Contre le Cancer) has suggested a classification based on tumour size (T), node status (N), and whether the cancer has spread to form a secondary tumour (metastasis) elsewhere (M). The stage (as described above) is a combination of node status and whether or not there are secondary tumours. The TNM classification can be applied to all cancers; you may find it used in the department where you are treated.

Oestrogen receptor (ER) status

Some breast cancers require oestrogen for their continued growth and spread. They have many receptors for oestrogen (see Chapter 1) and are termed ER-positive. They tend to be less aggressive than those that are ER-negative, and survival is better.

Postmenopausal women are more likely to have ER-positive cancers, and after surgery will generally be prescribed hormone therapy, usually the anti-oestrogen Tamoxifen. Because it also has some action on ER-negative cancers, Tamoxifen is usually given to all postmenopausal patients. Premenopausal women are more likely to have post-operative chemotherapy, which has been shown to be better than Tamoxifen in this age-group, even for ER-positive cancers.

In this country not all breast units measure ER status. Medical lawsuits are much more common in the USA and part of the reason for carrying out ER measurement there is to avoid litigation. Most specialists in the UK consider that all postmenopausal patients should be treated with Tamoxifen, which is a relatively safe drug with few serious side-effects, whether their tumours are ER-positive or not. They therefore feel that ER measurements are unnecessary and a waste of valuable resources. Pooling of data from worldwide studies has shown a reduction in mortality of up to 25% in women treated post-operatively with Tamoxifen, as well as a reduction in second breast cancers.

Age

Women under the age of 35 are more liable to have ER-negative tumours, and tend to do worse than older women with similar types of tumour. They are therefore likely to be offered more intensive chemotherapy (see Chapter 9).

Other prognostic indicators

Chromosomes are coils of DNA (deoxyribonucleic acid) which contain the millions of genes which direct every activity of the body. Inside the nucleus of each normal cell there are 46 chromosomes – half derived from the mother and half from the father. Cancer cells may have too many or too few chromosomes. This is called their ploidy. The nearer to normal, the better the prognosis. Scientists are also investigating whether the presence or increase in certain genes, receptors or enzymes indicates a worse prognosis.

Though all these measurements may be valuable in the future, at the present time the size of the tumour, tumour grade and node status are by far the most useful.

What about my cancer?

Statistics are useful when applied to large numbers of people. If we study 1,000 women with breast cancer, about 620 will be alive five years after diagnosis. Even if some of the good and bad cases came in clusters, the large numbers would even out the final result. If we study only ten women, more than six out of ten may survive – if the group contains a cluster of women with small, well-differentiated tumours that have not spread to the nodes. Conversely, the ten may contain a cluster of bad prognosis patients.

It is therefore not possible to know what the future holds for any individual patient, but if you want to know what your chances are the specialist can give you some indication. However, it will still only be a guide, as people are very unpredictable. Although patients with Stage 4 cancers usually don't do very well, some will survive ten years or more. Conversely, a small proportion of women with what appears to be Stage 1 (localized) cancer will die of their disease.

Types of breast cancer

It used to be thought that some breast cancers were derived from cells in the ducts (ductal carcinomas) and some from cells in the lobules (lobular carcinomas). It is now considered that they all arise from the TDLU (terminal duct lobular unit – see Chapter 1, especially Figure 2, p. 6), though the names for the two main forms seen under the microscope are still used. By far the most frequent breast cancers are ductal carcinomas; a smaller number are lobular carcinomas.

Less common carcinomas include medullary, tubular, colloid and cystic cancers of various kinds: these four types have a particularly good prognosis and a low chance of spreading to form secondary cancers elsewhere.

Inflammatory cancer is an uncommon breast cancer that makes the skin hot and red above it. It grows quickly and women with this type may not do well. However, after you've felt your lump again and again to make sure it's really there, your breast may be red and sore. This does not mean you have a cancer of this type, or that you have cancer at all. Only a specialist can make the diagnosis with certainty.

Other malignant tumours

Much less frequently tumours arise from the connective tissue, fat or overlying skin instead of from the breast tissue itself. The rare, giant version of a fibroadenoma is called cystosarcoma phyllodes, or phyllodes tumour. It is usually a tumour of fairly low malignancy.

Paget's disease of the nipple

Sometimes there are cancer cells in the skin around the nipple in a condition which resembles eczema. This is called Paget's disease, and it is almost always accompanied by a cancer within the breast tissue as well.

Bilateral and multiple cancers

Cancer can occur in both breasts, and is then called bilateral cancer. The tumours may be discovered at the same time, or a cancer may be found in the second breast several years later. If you have had one breast cancer you are more likely to develop cancer in the other breast. Your other breast will therefore be examined at follow-up visits, and regular mammograms taken. Lobular carcinomas are more likely than ductal carcinomas to occur on both sides.

When a pathologist examines the whole of a breast removed for cancer, every now and again he discovers one or more tiny cancers, quite separate from the main tumour. Recurrence in the breast is more likely after lumpectomy than after mastectomy because these tiny tumours may be present in the breast tissue which is left behind. Most surgeons therefore recommend radiotherapy after lumpectomy, to kill off any of these minute cancers.

It can be very disheartening to find that, after all, you need to have a mastectomy if the cancer recurs, so some women choose to have a mastectomy on being told about the possibility of recurrence. However, if you do have to have mastectomy some time after you have been treated by lumpectomy, it does not affect your chances of survival.

Breast cancer during pregnancy and breast-feeding

Breast cancer during pregnancy or breast-feeding is unusual. Only about 3% of all breast cancers are diagnosed at this time, usually in women in their 30s. However, as more women delay having babies until their 40s, when breast cancer becomes more common (see Chapter 3), more cancers may be discovered during pregnancy.

During pregnancy the breasts are enlarged and often tender, but persistent lumps should not be ignored. Go and see your doctor if you are worried. You should continue to examine your breasts during pregnancy, and breast-examination by the doctor should be part of antenatal care. If a lump is found, it is safe to perform an FNA or take a sample (biopsy – see Chapter 6) under local anaesthetic, and a general anaesthetic is safe after the first three months. The majority of lumps found in the breast during pregnancy or breast-feeding are benign. If the tests show that the lump is definitely benign, surgery can delayed until after the baby's birth.

It used to be thought that breast cancer during pregnancy resulted in serious consequences for both the mother and the pregnancy. However, although it is tragic to find you have cancer at this time, the outlook is the same as for other women with cancers of the same stage. A woman does not have to decide whether to continue with the pregnancy on the grounds of safety to either herself or her baby. There are no reported cases in which breast cancer has spread to a baby in the womb.

However, it is not desirable for a woman to take anti-cancer drugs during pregnancy, in case the drugs affect the baby. Labour can be induced when the baby is sufficiently mature, so if you decide to continue with your pregnancy, it may be possible to postpone chemotherapy until after the baby is born. You will be advised to stop breast-feeding if cancer is found after the baby is born and surgery is necessary. The increased blood supply to the breast during lactation makes surgery more difficult.

Breast-feeding should also be stopped if chemotherapy is needed, since these drugs can pass into the milk.

Breast cancer is most likely to recur or spread during the first few years. It is usually recommended that a woman should postpone having another baby for two to four years after surgery for breast cancer.

Breast cancer in men

By far the commonest cause of a breast lump in a man is gynaecomastia (see Chapter 2). Less than 1% of breast cancers occur in men, and there are only about 200 cases annually in the whole of the UK. Whereas breast cancer is most common in women in their 60s, in men it tends to occur about ten years later, among men in their 70s. Most are of the ductal type. The outcome for men and women is similar for the same type and stage of disease. However, men with breast cancer are more likely to wait before seeking treatment until the lump has broken through the skin to form an ulcer or become attached to the chest wall. While women think every breast lump must be cancer, men think a lump in the chest can't be cancer and may ignore it.

Primary, recurrent and secondary breast cancer

Primary breast cancer

The cancer you have in your breast is called a primary cancer. If you also develop cancer in the other breast, that is also a primary cancer, and you are said to have bilateral (primary) cancer.

Local recurrence

Local recurrence is when a tumour re-grows in or near the previous site. More commonly after lumpectomy than after mastectomy, a few cancer cells may be left behind and may grow into a new tumour. That is why lumpectomy is usually followed by radiotherapy, to kill off any cancer cells in the remaining breast tissue. Even after mastectomy, a tiny amount of breast tissue can remain behind. A tumour can therefore recur in the mastectomy scar.

If you notice a lump on or near the scar, see your doctor as soon as you find it. Sometimes scars heal a bit lumpily, and your doctor will be able to reassure you. If it is a recurrence, it can be treated. Don't leave it or it can develop into an ulcer that is more difficult to deal with.

Local spread

If breast cancer breaks through the overlying skin to form an open ulcer, or grows into the underlying chest muscle, this is called local spread. The cancer is still a primary cancer and it is classified as locally advanced cancer or Stage 3 disease. In the bad old days before radiotherapy and chemotherapy, when only radical mastectomy was on offer, many women put off seeing a doctor until they had extensive local spread. Even so, nearly 20% (one in five) survived five years.

Distant spread (secondary cancer)

Cancers can spread to other sites in the body via the lymphatics and the blood stream (see Chapter 3), or via body cavities like the minute space between the lungs and the chest wall (the pleural cavity). This is called distant spread. We now think that many, if not all, breast cancers (and other types of cancer) shed cells into these routes quite early on. Minute outposts of cancer cells form, which are not visible to the naked eye. Some lie dormant for many years before taking hold and growing into a secondary cancer. Many of them never develop any further, and are harmless. If cancer cells spread and grow to form tumours at sites away from the breast, these are called secondary tumours or secondary deposits or metastases.

The first place to which cancers of the breast usually spread is the lymphatic glands of the armpit (see Chapter 1). That is why doctors feel under your armpits to see if those glands are enlarged. The lymphatics of the breast also drain to the glands at the root of the neck, so that is another place which should be examined. If the glands are very large and hard, the doctor can be fairly certain they contain cancer deposits. To be certain he may need to remove some by an FNA (see Chapter 6). Removal of the lymph glands in the armpit (axillary clearance) is usually carried out as part of the operation for the removal of primary breast cancer. In the days of radical mastectomy and even more heroic operations, it was thought you could clear the underarm and other local lymph glands completely, and so halt the spread of cancer. We now know that this was a false hope; the operation is now carried out in order to tell whether cancer has spread to your lymph glands. If the lymph glands in your armpit contain cancer, this is called Stage 2 disease; but if they have become attached to the overlying skin or other tissues, this is Stage 3 advanced disease. If you have only one to four axillary lymph nodes containing cancer, you have almost as good a prognosis as if you had none.

If cancer spreads to your axillary lymph glands, you may notice that there is a lump in your armpit – or your arm on that side may swell (lymphoedema). Surgery or radiotherapy may also result in lymphoedema (see Chapter 8), and some people have lymphoedema due to causes other than cancer.

For reasons we don't understand, certain organs are preferred sites for cancers to spread to via the blood stream. In the case of breast cancer, the preferred sites are the liver, the lungs and their covering (the pleura), the bones and the brain. Part of the reason is that these are large organs, but some tissues like our muscles are equally large but are rarely the site of secondary cancer. Patients with deposits of cancer in these organs are Stage 4.

Having a secondary cancer in a bone is quite different from having primary bone cancer. The cells which have spread are like those in your primary breast cancer. They look like them under the microscope, behave like them and often respond to the same anti-cancer drugs. Similarly, a secondary cancer in your lung is not a lung cancer. It looks and behaves quite differently from a primary cancer of the lung.

5

Can I avoid breast cancer?

Risk factors and protective factors

A risk factor is something which increases the risk of a disease developing. If you go out in the cold and get soaking wet, you are more likely to catch a cold. Cold and wet are risk factors for the common cold. If you have a very pale skin, you are more at risk of getting severe sunburn than someone with a darker skin. Pale skin is a risk factor for sunburn, as well as for the most serious of skin cancers, melanomas. We take risk factors into consideration constantly in everyday life, weighing up the risks of doing something. Is it worth avoiding such risks, or would we rather take our chances? If it is pouring with rain, we can choose either to remain indoors and miss watching the rugby match, or to go just the same. If we have a pale skin, we can stay out of the sun or use a high-factor sun cream.

At present, we just do not know what causes breast cancer or how to avoid it. There are some well-recognised risk factors, most of them outside our control. They include getting older, having a close female relative with cancer, starting periods early, having the menopause late, and having no children or having a first baby after the age of 35. The reverse reduces risk – starting periods late, having the menopause early, and having a first baby in our teens. Many of these factors are believed to be linked with the way our bodies handle the female sex hormone, oestrogen, and the exposure to it of our incompletely matured breasts. Although most women who develop breast cancer have none of the known risk factors, these factors may nevertheless give us a clue as to its prevention.

Statistics and stories

It has been suggested, but never proved beyond doubt, that obesity, for example, is a risk factor in breast cancer. To prove it beyond doubt, it would have to be shown that the different rates of occurrence of breast cancer in women who are very overweight and those who are not, could not be by chance. If the difference is very small, it could have occurred by chance, and it is said not to be statistically significant. The findings are therefore called 'anecdotal' – a story (see Chapter 3). A doctor may have the impression that women with breast cancer are usually overweight.

This could have occurred by chance if his practice were in a part of the country where women tend to be on the plump side. It is often difficult to remain objective about impressions. New ideas are often picked up and 'hyped' by the media, and doctors have to guard against jumping to conclusions based on a small number of patients.

Age

Except for those few cancers which occur more commonly in the young (like tumours of muscle or bone), the older you are the more likely you are to get cancer, as shown in Figure 6. It is unusual to develop breast cancer before the age of 25, though rarely it occurs in little girls. As our expectation of life increases, so does our chance of getting cancer somewhere, but provided it can be diagnosed and treated successfully, we can still live to a ripe, old age.

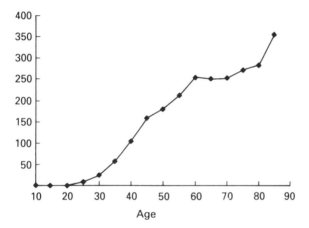

Figure 6 New cases of breast cancer at different ages (per 100,000 women)

Close relative with breast cancer

A very small number of women with breast cancer belong to cancer-prone families. Having a mother, sister or aunt who had breast cancer increases your risk. This risk is greater if their cancer was bilateral (in both breasts) or occurred before the menopause.

A gene is the unit of DNA in the chromosome of a cell that determines an aspect of how a cell behaves. Sometimes a change in a gene, called a mutation, is unimportant – for example, a change in the gene that controls hair or eye colour. However, if the change makes the cell more likely to get out of control and keep dividing to form a cancer, this is a serious change. Less than 5% of breast cancer patients come from families where the control genes are always defective. In these people cancer is more likely to develop, sometimes in one organ and sometimes in several. These families also have an unusually high incidence of cancers of the ovary, large bowel and prostate. For women belonging to some breast cancer families, there is about an 85% chance of developing breast cancer.

One advantage of identifying the gene defect is that those women who possess the faulty gene can be warned that they are at risk, and those who do not can be reassured. However, the psychological effects of the knowledge can be very profound, and are the subject of concern to health professionals. Detecting these abnormal genes, such as *BRCA1* and *BRCA2*, is still a research technique, and not available generally.

Women from such families should have a baseline mammogram from the age of 30 or 35, to have a record of how their normal breast appears. It has been recommended that they have regular examination, with mammograms five-yearly till the age of 40, then every two years until they are 50, when it has been recommended they have annual mammograms, with surgery if and when a lump is found. Some women at high risk have decided to have bilateral mastectomy and immediate breast reconstruction (see Chapter 10), even before a tumour has been diagnosed.

Studies are planned to see whether taking the anti-oestrogen Tamoxifen will prevent women at high risk from getting breast cancer. Animal experiments suggest that human chorionic gonadotrophin (HCG – a hormone produced by the placenta during pregnancy) might protect against breast cancer. This would make the breasts mature completely, as they do at the end of the first pregnancy. Scientists are also working towards being able to treat defective genes by synthesizing substances to counter their actions, or by injecting genes directly into the cancer.

Oncogenes and tumour suppressor genes

It was thought there were specific genes, called oncogenes, which caused cancer. We now realize that most of these are normal genes which have been damaged by ultraviolet light, substances in cigarette smoke, pollutants and so on.

Some genes, such as *p53*, are necessary for the control of normal growth, to stop us all becoming giants. They also act to stop tumours developing, and are therefore called tumour suppressor genes. When these genes are damaged, some of the molecules of which they are formed are changed (mutated) into similar but abnormal ones. The changed gene no longer works as a policeman to stop cells becoming malignant: 5% of patients with breast cancer have been found to have mutations in one or more tumour suppressor genes.

The oestrogen window

During the first two weeks of each monthly period we produce a surge of unopposed oestrogen – that is, oestrogen without progesterone. The 'oestrogen window' is the gap between the time when the breasts start to develop at puberty and when they become fully mature at the end of the first pregnancy. The breasts are thought to be particularly vulnerable to cancer-producing influences (carcinogens) during this time.

Age at first period (menarche), and age at menopause

Those who start their periods before the age of 12, or undergo their menopause after 55, or have more than 40 years of menstrual cycles, are at greater risk of breast cancer. In primitive peoples, where women go from one pregnancy to the next, menstruation occurs infrequently – perhaps only 40 times in all, compared with 400 times for women in developed countries. In some Western countries the average age of the first period has gone down to 10 or 11. This is thought to be due to improvement in our diet generally, and to an increase in fat in our diet in particular. In developing countries, menstruation may not start until 17 or 18, with a first pregnancy following soon afterwards.

The improved diet and earlier onset of periods also result in women being taller, and there is a suggestion that taller women have higher rates of breast cancer.

Women who have had their ovaries removed for any reason (such as cysts on both ovaries) before the age of 35, and so have an artificially early menopause, have a lower incidence of breast cancer.

Pregnancy and breast-feeding

Having a first full-term pregnancy when young helps protect against breast cancer. Conversely, having a first baby after the age of 35, or having no children at all, increases the risk of breast cancer. Women are tending to postpone having children until their careers are established. Not only do we have more periods because we start earlier, but the time from our first period to the first full-term pregnancy is longer. The pregnancy must be full-term for it to have a protective effect; miscarriages do not do this. It is not until the end of pregnancy that the breast fully matures and becomes less vulnerable.

Breast-feeding probably needs to be carried out for a total of two years in all to have a protective effect, and many women breast-feed for considerably less than this. There are, of course, many advantages for the breast-fed baby: the mother's immunity is transferred to the baby in her breast milk, particularly in the thick colostrum produced in the first few days of breast-feeding; breast-fed babies also have a lower incidence of gastro-intestinal and other infections.

Benign breast disease

Benign breast disease does not increase the risk of cancer, unless you also have a family history of breast cancer or your breast lump contains atypical (cancer-like) cells (see Chapter 2). In this group, much more careful follow-up is therefore required. Some women who have had several benign lumps in which atypical cells were found have opted for mastectomy, rather than go on worrying about whether they might later develop cancer.

Previous cancer in the other breast or uterus

The influences which cause breast cancer affect the body as a whole, and both breasts. If you have had one breast cancer, you have an increased risk of developing a second. Women are carefully followed up and have regular mammography, so that if a second cancer develops it can be dealt with while still very small. Cancer of the uterus is also influenced by sex hormones, and breast cancer is more frequent in women who have also had cancer of the endometrial lining of the uterus.

Obesity and high blood-levels of insulin

The hormone insulin controls blood-sugar levels. Some obese women who put on weight round their middles – 'apples' rather than 'pears' – have high blood-levels of insulin and an insulin-like growth factor. Both of these substances are involved in breast development and may increase the risk of breast cancer. They may also have high levels of the male hormone, testosterone, which can be converted to oestrogen in fat (see Chapter 1), so fat women tend to have more available oestrogen. The interaction of obesity and breast cancer is under study in a number of centres, but whether the fashionable image is slim or plump, being overweight certainly increases the risk of heart disease.

The contraceptive pill

Most studies show that there is probably no increased risk of cancer with modern, low-dose combined oestrogen and progesterone pills, but the early, high-dose oestrogen pills were thought to increase the risk slightly. Progesterone-only pills appear to have no effect on the occurrence of breast cancer. It has been claimed that the Pill reduces benign breast disease, but this may just mean that women on the Pill have less cyclical breast pain and so consult their GPs less.

There is concern about young girls being on the Pill for prolonged periods of time while their breasts are developing. As yet, there is no evidence to suggest that the incidence of breast cancer will increase when they reach the age at which cancer becomes more common. The fact that unwanted pregnancies and abortions have their own risks, and a small but real mortality, is used as an argument to support the continued use of the Pill for the young.

Hormone replacement therapy (HRT)

There is a slightly higher risk of breast cancer in women who have had hormone replacement therapy (HRT). Some would argue that the improvement in menopausal symptoms (such as vaginal dryness and hot flushes), and in reducing heart disease, osteoporosis and possibly Alzheimer's disease, more than make up for any increase in the risk of breast cancer. This is something each woman must decide for herself. It is probably unwise to continue on HRT for more than 10–15 years. If there is a family history of breast cancer, some specialists would advise against HRT.

Irradiation

Women whose breasts were exposed to irradiation, especially between the ages of 10 and 14 when their breasts were developing, are at greater risk of cancer. These include Japanese women who survived the atom bombs, and women treated for various medical conditions by irradiation. Before we had specific treatment for tuberculosis, patients were repeatedly examined under X-ray. The present view is that an occasional chest X-ray is unlikely to be dangerous – and the possible adverse effect of the very small dose of X-rays required for mammography is more than outweighed by the benefit of detecting breast cancer early. We do not yet know to what extent nuclear accidents like that at Chernobyl and elsewhere may contribute to breast cancer incidence.

Alcohol

Several studies have now shown an increased risk of breast cancer in women who drink as little as two alcoholic drinks a day, of whatever type. Alcohol attacks liver cells, and alcoholics can develop, and even die of, cirrhosis of the liver. Women have a higher risk of liver damage than men, and the oestrogens which are normally broken down by the healthy liver accumulate and increase the risk of breast cancer. You have to weigh this against the suggestion that a small amount of alcohol helps to protect against heart disease.

Diet

It has been suggested that the difference between the incidence of breast cancer in Europe and the USA compared with Japan is because we eat more animal fat, and that certain dietary fats help cancers to spread. When Japanese women emigrate to the USA and adopt a Western diet, the number of cases of breast cancer increases. However, Japanese-Americans with breast cancer live longer than white Americans with the same disease, so other factors are also important, such as their way of life, or other aspects of diet. Some types of fat and fish-oils are protective but it may be the extra calories that are important. If animal fats were the most important factor, reduced rates of breast cancer should be seen in vegetarians – but this has not been found to be the case.

Results from experiments in rats are quite clear. Rates of breast cancer induced in rats are much higher in those on a high-fat diet. No such proof exists in humans. One possibility is that women are so different from rats that the results are not comparable. Another suggestion is that it is easier to control exactly what rats are given to eat. Prospective or retrospective studies require women to record or remember what type and quantity of food they have eaten. If you have ever tried to diet by counting calories you will know how easy it is to forget what you have eaten that day – let alone last year.

Socio-economic status

Affluent women are more likely to get cancer than their poorer sisters. This is thought to be due to a combination of diet (higher both in calories and in animal fat), and of later first full-term pregnancy.

Stress and personality

The effects of stress and personality type are extremely difficult to measure. When any of us develops breast cancer we immediately wonder what caused it, and it is easy to magnify stressful events which we would otherwise have taken in our stride. There is no doubt that our modern Western life-style is stressful. However, the Japanese (for example) are also subject to stress, and they have one of the lowest rates of breast cancer in the world. Studies following up groups of people seem to suggest that those who are highly stressed and unable to 'let it out' are more likely to develop cancer. However, before the discovery of the tubercle bacillus, there was thought to be a tuberculosis-prone type – sensitive and poetic. We now know that the most important factor is the dose of TB bacteria.

Stress can be shown to lower immunity, and so may act by reducing the body's natural ability to seek out and destroy abnormal cells before they become cancerous. Furthermore, if we are stressed we may consume more alcohol or eat for comfort, increasing our cancer risk in that way.

One of the problems in examining the effect of stress is that a cancer one centimetre in diameter (about the size of your thumbnail, or a bit less) contains one billion cancer cells. Even if it is a fast-growing cancer, it will take up to ten years to reach that size. How many of us can recall all of the stressful events which happened years before? Mostly when we look at our lives and wonder whether a major upset was responsible, we think in terms of two or three years. However, for some people most events are stressful, while others are able to take even major disasters in their stride.

Pollution, pesticides and chemical by-products

The pollution to which we are all exposed, and the pesticides used in farming, would seem likely contributory factors to breast cancer. In Israel, banning a certain pesticide reduced breast cancer incidence, though this work has to be confirmed elsewhere. Some chemical by-products have an oestrogen-like action and may therefore stimulate breast cancers. There is pressure by a number of groups to investigate the effect of pollution by a variety of substances and agents.

Men and breast cancer

We know less about the causes of breast cancer in men. They too can belong to cancer-prone families. Some have been treated with female hormones, and some have been over-exposed to irradiation.

Unrelated factors

The following factors are not presently thought to be associated with breast cancer.

Tea and coffee drinking

Early studies seemed to suggest that coffee and tea drinking might be risk factors for breast cancer. However, when age of first pregnancy was taken into consideration, it became clear there was no such association. In countries where there has been a marked increase in coffee consumption and then a decrease there has been no corresponding change in the number of breast cancer cases.

Vitamins

Some studies suggest that groups of people who do not develop cancer have a high intake of beta carotene (a substance converted into vitamin A in the body), vitamins C, D and E, and the metal selenium. There is as yet no convincing evidence that adding any of these to the diet reduces the likelihood of breast cancer. Large studies are in progress to see whether they will do so.

Smoking

The general view is that, once other risk factors are taken into consideration, there seems to be no difference in the occurrence of breast cancer between smokers and non-smokers. One of the effects of smoking is to bring forward the age of menopause by about a year. It has therefore been suggested that the risk in smokers may be lower because they have an earlier menopause. However, a study from Denmark found that women who had smoked for 20 to 30 years had an increased risk of breast cancer, but other studies have shown no such increase.

The incidence of lung cancer is, however, vastly increased in women who smoke. In Scotland and the USA, lung cancer is now the most common cancer in women, with breast cancer coming second.

Blows to the breast

Blows and minor injuries to your breast do not cause cancer. Rubbing the spot which has been knocked probably just draws attention to a lump which is already there. Injury (trauma) can cause some of the fat cells in the breast to die – this is called fat necrosis – and a hard scar may form. This can be mistaken for cancer (see Chapter 2), but it is not cancer, and it does not lead to cancer.

Wearing bras

There has been a recent suggestion, not published in the medical press, that wearing bras – especially at night – is a risk factor for breast cancer. This is not generally accepted.

Non-breast cancer in other members of the family

While having a close relative with breast cancer increases your risk, having a relative with cancer in other organs, such as the lung or bowel, has no such effect, except in the very small number of families with defective genes (see above).

Myths

There are many misconceptions about cancer, which the following may help to dispel.

- **Cancer is not one disease.** Cancers can arise in any organ of the body and there are over 200 different types, with different causes and requiring different treatment. Each organ is made of several tissues. The breast, for example, contains milk-producing breast tissue, fat, connective (supporting) tissue, muscle and blood vessels and is covered by skin. Tumours can develop from any one of these, although in the breast, cancers most commonly arise from the terminal duct lobular units (TDLUs, see Chapter 1).

- **Breast cancer is not your fault.** We look at risk factors to try to find *why* breast cancer develops, but most women have none of these factors. In my view, it is downright wicked to teach that if you have breast cancer you are responsible, and that if you had taken enough thought you could have prevented it. Lung cancer is different: the evidence that smoking is the prime cause in the West is beyond doubt and every packet of cigarettes carries a health warning. There is no such clear-cut cause of breast cancer.

- **Cancer is not a punishment.** It's natural to wonder why it has happened to you and to feel it must be your fault. When we are told we have breast cancer, we all wonder, 'Why me? What did I do or not do? Am I being punished for some real or imagined wickedness?' Saints and sinners alike develop cancer. Women in the UK have a lifetime risk of 1 in 12 of getting breast cancer. It is impossible to believe breast cancer only occurs in the wicked minority, and that the rest are angels.

- **Breast cancer is not caused by sexual promiscuity or related to it in any way.** Often women try to think back to any indiscretion, and worry that they have brought their cancer on themselves by misbehaving.

- **Cancer of the breast cannot be caught or induced by reading about it.** Some people avoid friends with cancer because they feel they do not know how to approach the subject and feel embarrassed, but a few believe they can catch it. Some women are afraid even to read about cancer, because they feel in some way that thinking, talking or reading about breast cancer will make them develop it. In mice it seems that there is a cancer virus which can be passed to the litter in the mother's milk. In humans there are a few cancers thought to be caused by viruses – for example, cervical and liver cancer, and these viruses are passed from person to person. Every now and again, someone 'discovers' a human breast cancer virus, but at the moment (1996) there is no concrete evidence of a viral cause of human breast cancer.

So how can we avoid breast cancer?

At this stage in our knowledge, there is little positive that we can positively do to avoid breast cancer. We cannot choose the age at which we start having periods, nor when we experience the menopause. Few of us would make the decision on when or whether to have children based on the risk of getting breast cancer. We can, however, choose a lower-fat diet, drink little if any alcohol, and avoid getting overweight.

We can also make sure that the cancer is treated when it is small. In the UK, about 80% of all cancers are found by the woman or her partner. GPs do not routinely examine every woman's breast when she comes for a check-up. Furthermore the percentage of women turning up for free NHS mammography offered from the age of 50 is nothing like as high in this country as it is, for example, in Scandinavia. In the UK the uptake overall is about 70%, but in inner city areas it is as low as 60%. In countries with an uptake of 80–90% there has been a marked decrease in the size and stage of the cancers seen, with a corresponding decrease in deaths from breast cancer.

We can make sure that we, or our GP, examine our breasts regularly. If we find a lump, we can go at once to the doctor instead of delaying. In this country nearly two thirds of women with breast cancer do survive. This figure is even higher in countries where breast cancers are detected earlier.

This is something positive we can do while experts seek for new information on how to prevent breast cancer, and investigate new ways to treat it. Breast cancer is uncommon under the age of 25. From this age, women should examine their breasts regularly for lumps (see Chapter 6) and report anything suspicious to their GP. Pain and lumpiness are common before a period, but lumps which persist throughout the cycle should be taken seriously. The incidence of breast cancer increases with age, and mammography is offered free to all women over 50 through the NHS. Any woman with a near relative who has had breast cancer needs to be extra vigilant.

The role of diet in breast cancer is unproven, but the present view is that a healthy diet boosts your immune system and may help to prevent cancer. You should eat less fat, cut down on sugar, eat more vegetables, fruit and cereals, and reduce the amount of salt to help prevent heart disease.

Some women have gone to extremes, going back to the bad old days when we were all pressurized to marry early and bear lots of children, and exert unfair pressure on their daughters. Women who have their first baby later in life do have a greater risk of breast cancer. It would, however, require very large studies to prove that *changing* our social habits would reduce the risk of breast cancer. Such studies do not exist.

6

Diagnosis

Diagnosis is the medical term for finding out the exact nature of what is wrong with you. Breast cancer may be diagnosed by the doctor examining you, or your mammogram, or cells from a fine needle aspirate (see p. 58), or a portion of your lump. Unlike cancer of the lung or bowel or other vital organs, breast cancer doesn't make you feel ill or lose weight, and most are not painful. Unless you have your breasts examined, or have a mammogram, you may not know anything is wrong.

Breast Awareness

The emphasis nowadays is on *breast awareness*. This means knowing what your breasts are normally like so you can spot any change in how they look or feel.

Women need to be told that breast cancer is not necessarily a death sentence. In the UK, more than six out of ten women with breast cancer will survive at least five years, more if the tumour is small and has not yet spread. Most breast lumps are found by women or their partners – but too many women purposely delay going to their doctor for months or even years.

From the age of 50 in the UK you will receive invitations to three-yearly mammography, but you should still examine your own breasts. Never ignore a lump, whatever your age. Doctors would far rather you came to see them with something benign, or because you are worried, than that you ignore a cancer. If you are worried and your GP is dismissive, be persistent, or change to a more sympathetic one.

Most women's breasts are a bit swollen and lumpy in the second half of the menstrual cycle, so examine your breasts soon after a period when they are softest. It used to be recommended that premenopausal women regularly examine their breasts after each period, and that after the menopause, women should examine their breasts on a certain day of each calendar month. If this suits you it is a good idea; but opinion has swung against a rigid timetable, since studies did not show that Breast Self Examination (BSE) reduced mortality. However, if it picked up cancers when they were small enough to be removed by lumpectomy instead of mastectomy, it would still be worthwhile. Examine your breasts when you are relaxed – not when you are tearing off to work or hurrying to get the shopping.

You should get to know your breasts, how they look and how they feel. Don't worry if one is bigger than the other, or that the nipples aren't level. This is normal. What you are looking for are *changes*. Get used to having a good look at your breasts in front of the mirror, first with your hands by your sides and then with them above your head. Place your hands on your hips and press your shoulders inwards to make your chest muscles tighten.

Feel your breasts using a soapy hand in the bath or shower. Pay special attention to the upper, outer area, where 60% of breast cancers occur. If you have large breasts you may find it easier lying down. Feel the right breast with the left hand, and vice versa. Use the flat of your hand and don't prod or squeeze. If you always have lumpy breasts, look for changes. Move your hand round the edge of your breasts and then round the centre. Feel behind your nipple, up into your armpit and towards your collar bone. If you are worried, go and see your GP right away.

The risk of breast cancer increases with age, but some older women are embarrassed to feel their breasts. They should remember that if they find a cancer when it is small, they have a much better chance of living to be a hundred! If you do find a lump, you will be feeling some surrounding tissue with it: the actual tumour will almost certainly be much smaller than the lump you can feel.

We need to feel that examining our breasts for changes is no different from looking at our nails to see if they need filing, or at our legs to see whether they need waxing. We need to know that if we do find a lump, we will be examined sympathetically and treated quickly and efficiently. Above all, more publicity needs to be given to the good outlook for breast cancer compared with most other cancers. The death-rate from breast cancer is finally falling in all but the oldest women.

If you come from a breast cancer family (see Chapter 5), you may already have received counselling about the need to have regular check-ups. Some experts recommend that your breasts should be examined by a doctor once you have reached the age of 30, when you should have a 'baseline' mammogram to show what your breast is like normally. This will enable the radiologist to look for changes when you start having regular mammograms.

Changes to look out for:

- lumps or swellings in your breast or armpit;
- changes in the shape or size of your breast;
- discharge or bleeding from your nipple; a rash on or around it; moist, reddish areas that do not heal;
- change in the position of your nipple – inverted (pulled inwards) if it used to stick out, or pointing in a different direction;

- dimples, dents or fine pitting (orange-peel appearance);
- pain in your breast which is new for you;
- swelling of your arm;
- prominent veins on your breast.

Screening

Screening is the investigation of apparently healthy people for a condition that they are unaware of having. We are all used to being screened. We are asked for a specimen of urine when we have a medical for insurance purposes, join a new GP practice, or go to an antenatal clinic. The urine specimen is tested for sugar to see whether we have diabetes, even though we have no signs or symptoms of that disease.

Symptoms are what we complain of, like pain or feeling tired. *Signs* are those things which can be seen, felt or measured by another person. Some symptoms are also signs. You may, for example, go to your GP because you have felt a lump in your breast which is sometimes tender and sometimes not. This is your main symptom. Your GP will be able to feel the lump, so it is both a symptom and a sign. If you go on a day when it is tender, he will be able to tell that it hurts when he touches it, so tenderness can also be a sign. If you go on a day when it is not tender, he will have to take your word that it is painful. In this case pain is a symptom not a sign.

Mammography and mammograms

A mammogram is a low-dose X-ray which can show up the minute specks of calcium that are formed in many breast cancers, as well as other changes in the breast. Tiny cancers less than half a centimetre in diameter can be identified by this technique. These would be much too small to be felt, even by the most experienced doctor. Previously, these minute tumours were only found by chance when lumps were removed from the breast for other reasons (fibrocystic change, for example – see Chapter 2). After removal of a breast lump, you always have to wait a few days for the result, because it takes time for the pathologist to process and report on all the tissue removed.

Breast screening

In 1991 a nation-wide service of three-yearly mammography for all women between 50 and 64 was set up in the UK. Mammography picks up more cancers when they are small enough to be removed by lumpectomy – and in addition, some studies have shown a 40% drop in deaths from breast cancer as a result of the screening programme. If you are over 50, you should have been sent an appointment, provided your GP has your correct address. He will be able to arrange for you to have a mammogram if you are between 50 and 64 and somehow got missed, or if you are over 64 and wish to have one.

It seems difficult to believe that at present women over 64 are not invited to have regular mammograms, given that the risk of breast cancer increases with age. Many women over the age of 64 are fit and well, and deserve early treatment as much as younger women. It seems unlikely that cost implications would be considered important if the suggestion were to stop screening for prostate or colon cancer in men over the age of 64. In some districts, 80% of women sent appointments have come for screening – but the figure is as low as 60% in some inner city areas. The excuse that even fewer women over 64 would respond has been used to justify excluding them. I know some of the reasons why older women might not attend, though most women have no problems at all.

> I was sent an appointment to attend a mobile unit miles away, because the part of London where I live had been taken over by another NHS district. It was not possible for me to go to the nearby centre because of the difficulty of cross-invoicing between districts. Instructions on how to get there by bus were included with the invitation, but none of the buses went anywhere near where I live, and there was no information on getting there by Underground. A hand-drawn map showing the position of the mobile unit was faint and hard to read. Had I been a little old lady (as I am), and not used to finding my way to faraway places, I might easily have been another 'non-attender'.
>
> I live within walking distance of several hospitals. When I telephoned the screening centre, I was offered an alternative appointment at a hospital the other side of London, or in Middlesex, a railway journey away! However, the two radiographers couldn't have been nicer or more professional (I didn't let on until afterwards that I was a doctor).
>
> I sympathized with my friends who felt embarrassed at going up the steps to the mobile unit in a supermarket car-park, with everyone watching. They much preferred it when the unit was situated in hospital grounds.

At the mammography unit

Your visit shouldn't take more than about half-an-hour. Don't use a deodorant, creams or talcum powder on that day – they may show up on the film and make the mammogram difficult to interpret. You will need to undress to the waist, so it is best to wear separates. The radiographer will compress each breast in turn between rigid plastic plates. It always hurts to have your breasts squeezed hard, but it is soon over. Whenever I have a mammogram, I always expect it to be worse than it is. Remember to warn the radiographer if you have had a breast implant (see Chapter 10).

Jennifer's breasts had been enlarged by silicone implants some years before, when she was working as a model. The result was so good you couldn't tell, and she had told no-one about her operation. She didn't tell the radiographer who had trouble getting a good picture until she realized the reason. Jennifer was a bit upset to find you could tell – even though you needed an X-ray machine to do so!

Finding out your results

After your mammogram, you will be told approximately when you will get your results – it should be within three weeks. If the mammograms are not satisfactory for technical reasons, you may be asked to come back to have them taken again. This does not necessarily mean there is an abnormality.

If there is an area on the mammogram that looks unusual, you will be sent an appointment for an assessment clinic at a hospital. There you will be seen by a doctor, and you may need further mammograms. If an abnormality is confirmed, you will be referred to the most convenient hospital breast clinic. The proportion of women needing to have their mammography repeated is highest in the 50–54 age group, because it is more difficult to interpret mammograms in younger women. The doctor may decide to draw off some cells for examination under the microscope, guided by what can be seen on the mammogram. This is called a stereotactic fine needle aspirate (FNA).

The pros and cons of mammography

Some studies have shown up to a 40% decrease in deaths from breast cancer when 80–90% of women have come forward for mammography. However, women may go through unnecessary anxiety because of small abnormalities – which may never have progressed and which are now found and operated on. Another disadvantage is that X-rays are used, though the dose is small. Opponents also claim that, even if cancers are found, they may already have spread and the woman merely knows she has cancer for longer.

However, nearly half the cancers picked up by mammography screening are less than one centimetre in diameter. Cancers of this size are less likely to have spread to lymph nodes or elsewhere in the body, and the outlook is excellent. Whether they have spread or not, the primary breast cancer can be removed without the surgeon having to remove the whole breast. Many experts consider the risk of the small dose of X-rays negligible compared with the value of picking up breast cancer before it has spread.

Some of the controversy concerning mammography has been published, and some well-known figures consider it a waste of public money. If there was any chance of there being a small cancer in my breast – or anywhere else for that matter – I would want it out NOW. I wouldn't want to take a chance on it being a good cancer which isn't going to grow and spread. As far as I am concerned, the only good cancer is one that is dead and in a specimen pot full of formaldehyde, or one that has just been removed and is about to be used for research.

Negative mammogram results and interval cancers

Like other medical tests, mammography is not 100% accurate, and cancers may not show up. If you find anything in your breast which worries you, go and see your doctor – even if you have had a recent mammogram reported as negative.

Recent studies have suggested that mammography should be carried out at two-yearly intervals rather than three-yearly, since a number of cancers (called interval cancers) become evident during the third year. The fact that so many interval cancers appear in the UK is some evidence that we have an aggressive type of breast cancer. It may take time for the Government to accept the cost of two-yearly mammography. It does mean we should not be complacent just because we have had a negative mammogram, but should continue to be breast aware.

Screening and Government targets

In its document *The Health of the Nation*, the Government pledged to reduce the number of deaths from breast cancer by at least 25% in women invited for screening by the year 2000. This is the group of women over 50 years old, in whom 80% of breast cancers presently occur. If breast cancers are identified when they are small and before they have spread, treatment is more likely to cure. It is hoped to save some 1,250 deaths per year, so the rate would drop from 95.1 per 100,000 of the female population to no more than 71.3 per 100,000. The rate has already fallen from 98.3 per 100,000 in 1985, but this is unlikely yet to be due to screening. In the year 1991–92, the screening programme detected 6,605 cancers which were completely unsuspected by the patient. Of these, 1,468 (24%) were one centimetre or less, a size which seldom results in death from breast cancer.

Aims in breast cancer screening and treatment

The Government has established target standards for breast cancer care:

- at least 70% of the women invited should attend for breast mammography;
- a maximum two week gap for 90% of women between the initial mammogram and recall for further tests;
- at least half the cancers detected should be 1.5 centimetres or less when detected. In this country, far too many cancers are first treated when they are much bigger, reducing the chance of cure;
- every woman with breast cancer should be told what options are available for her treatment, should be offered a choice where appropriate, and should be able to talk to a breast-care nurse;
- more than 50% of women with invasive cancers of 1.5 centimetres or less should be treated by lumpectomy;
- 90% of women should be admitted for surgery within two weeks of being told they need an operation.

Other types of tests

Ultrasound examination

Ultrasound examination is a technique whereby high frequency sound waves, too high to be heard by the human ear, are passed through the body. Distortions in the waves, caused by their passage through the tissues, are picked up by special recording equipment and converted into the ultrasound scans we are used to seeing of unborn babies in the womb. In younger women, with their denser breast tissue (see Chapter 1), ultrasound scans give a clearer picture than mammograms.

Jelly is rubbed over the breast and an ultrasound transmitter is rolled over it. A radiologist watches on the screen and takes permanent pictures as required. Other than being cold and sticky, it is a painless procedure.

Magnetic Resonance Imaging (MRI)

MRI scans create an image which looks rather like an X-ray; they are based mainly on differences in water-content between cancer and normal tissues. For this you lie on a table which is moved through a powerful magnetic field.

MRI has revolutionized the diagnosis and treatment of brain disease, and is particularly useful for looking at the brain to see whether secondary cancer is present. Some specialists in the USA have also been using MRI for breast cancer screening, but experts in the UK do not feel its value has been proved – and these scans are very expensive. However, since MRI scans do not use X-rays, they may prove useful in younger women at high risk, who would otherwise need repeated mammograms and repeated doses of X-rays.

CT scans

A CT scan (short for Computerised Axial Tomography) consists of a series of images taken while an X-ray camera moves over you. These are then assembled by computer.

Both CT scans and MRI scans take some time. Although they are painless, they can feel claustrophobic so you should be prepared for this.

Other types of scans

A bone scan, liver scan or brain scan may be necessary to check whether a cancer has spread. For a bone scan, a small amount of radioactive material is injected into a vein in your arm. An X-ray is taken up to one hour later, and any abnormal areas in your bones (including areas of osteoarthritis) show as 'hot spots'. Liver scans are carried out using ultrasound (see above) on the upper and mainly right hand side of your abdomen. Depending on circumstances, the doctor may order either a CT scan or an MRI scan of your brain.

Fine needle aspirate (FNA)

The surgeon (or a cytologist; see Chapter 7) may need to remove cells from your lump using a fine needle and a hypodermic syringe, and have the cells examined under the microscope. This process is called a fine needle aspirate (FNA), because the cells are aspirated (sucked up) into a syringe. It has the advantage that no anaesthetic is required, and the result can be available quickly. Having an FNA may be quite painless or very uncomfortable, depending on whether your lump is tender or not. There is nothing to suggest that malignant cells will spread along the needle track.

Biopsy

Although the surgeon may feel almost sure that the lump in your breast is cancer, the FNA results may not be conclusive. Cancer cells unfortunately don't have a big 'C' written on them – and distinguishing between slightly abnormal cells and cancer can be very difficult. The surgeon may therefore need to make certain of the diagnosis by removing a portion of your lump. This is called a biopsy.

There are three main ways of getting a sample of your lump to examine under the microscope:

- a small core of tissue can be removed under local anaesthetic using a hollow needle. This is called a *Tru-cut biopsy.*
- if a bigger piece is needed, it is usually removed under general anaesthetic. This is an *incision biopsy.*
- the surgeon may decide to remove the whole lump. This is an *excision biopsy.* If cancer is present, you may need a larger operation to be sure that there is a good margin of normal tissue around it.

It normally takes a few days for the results to come through. You will be sent home and given an appointment to come back and see the surgeon to discuss the results and further treatment, if any.

Frozen sections

Before FNAs became widely accepted, surgeons used to take a biopsy under general anaesthetic and ask the pathologist to examine the piece immediately, while the patient was still asleep. Instead of waiting for the normal processing schedule, the piece was frozen with a freezing spray. If the report came back that the lump was malignant, the surgeon went on to carry out an immediate mastectomy. This meant that the patient went into the operation not knowing whether she would wake up with her breast removed.

Nowadays, surgeons usually have an FNA report saying whether the lump is cancer or not, though sometimes cancer may be present and missed by the needle. If, when the surgeon operates to remove the lump, he finds it looks like cancer, he can ask for an immediate frozen section. If it is benign, there is nothing further to do. If it is confirmed to be cancer, the wound is closed and the surgeon will discuss any further treatment when you are fully awake.

Even if the lump looks benign on frozen section, it still takes a few days for the biopsy specimen to be processed and examined thoroughly. The problem with frozen sections is the time the process takes: if cancer is present, a report can be given at once; but if the lump appears benign, every bit must be examined to be absolutely certain that no cancer is present. It is therefore not usually possible for the pathologist to issue a final report as soon as your operation is carried out.

In the UK most excision biopsies are carried out under general anaesthetic. In the USA, where the cost of general anaesthetics and hospital care is so high, biopsies are often performed under local anaesthetic.

7
Doctors and hospitals

Your first stop – the GP

Your GP may know you from previous visits, or you may never have had a day's illness in your life and hardly know him. Go and see him as soon as you think you have found something wrong. If it is nothing serious, he can reassure you; if he finds a lump or anything of concern he will refer you to hospital. The services provided by the NHS are there to be used. Don't feel you are wasting time asking about things that worry you. It is far better to find that there is nothing to worry about than to delay going to see your doctor. If he cannot find a lump, and you think you have found one, be persistent; ask to see a specialist. The Cancer Relief Macmillan Fund (see Useful addresses) has produced a directory of breast cancer centres available to all GPs. If you need to see a specialist, ask your GP to send you to a surgeon who specialises in the treatment of breast problems.

If you don't yet have a GP, your local library has a list of GPs in the area, or you can get a list from your local Family Health Services Authority (FHSA – their address is in the phone directory). Keep your GP informed of any change of address so that you will be invited for breast and cervical screening. If you move out of the district, register with a new doctor even if at the moment you are perfectly well. If you are not happy with your doctor, or you would rather have a woman GP, you can change. All you have to do is to ask the new doctor whether you can be taken on his or her list. You don't have to go and tell your previous GP your reasons.

Link workers and language problems

Some health authorities and GP practices have link workers, especially in districts where there are large ethnic groups. If you or someone you know has a language difficulty, ask if a link worker is available. The link worker can remain to interpret while the patient is being examined.

Your first hospital visit

You have seen your GP and he has given you a letter to take to the hospital, or you have been sent a hospital appointment following mammography. Breast clinics try to make appointments within a week to ten days. If there has been something in the media that sends lots of women to see their doctor, you may have to wait longer. If you are very worried, go and nag your doctor, and he can try to bring your appointment forward.

Take your husband, partner or a friend with you if they can take time off work. Whether your breast lump turns out to be cancer or not, it is a stressful experience and it may be difficult for you to take in what has been said. Some people recommend taking a tape recorder.

It is best to prepare yourself for a long wait. Hospital staff are making a real effort to overcome the problem of the endless waiting about in hospital clinics, but there's a long way to go. Assume you may have to give up a whole morning or afternoon. If you are seen on time, that's a bonus. More women complain about sitting waiting in a room full of worried women, with no-one telling them what's happening, than about anything else. You can almost see the cloud of worry hovering above their heads. A friend suggested it should be called the 'Worried Women Clinic'! Perhaps there should be a big notice saying: 'Nine out of ten of you won't have cancer' – but that wouldn't be good for the tenth woman, who will. It doesn't help to be unpleasant to the doctors or the nurses because you're fed up at being kept waiting – they are already stressed and doing their best, often under difficult conditions.

The examination

The surgeon or his registrar will have a letter from your GP outlining your problem, but they will probably want to ask you how it all began (your medical history). In a teaching unit you might be asked if a medical student may examine you (students are discussed later in this chapter). They will want to examine both breasts and, depending on what they find, possibly your armpits and tummy also.

You will be asked to undress in an examination room on your own or behind a screen; you will need to take off your blouse (or jumper) and bra. Wear clothes which are easy to take off. You always have a feeling you must hurry, and then you catch your ear-ring in a high-necked jumper and have to struggle to get it free. At my own hospital, everyone dealing with breast problems feels very strongly that, after an examination, patients should be allowed to get dressed in peace before further tests or their future treatment is discussed with them. Hopefully this courtesy will spread to all breast units.

Jane said 'Almost the worst thing was being told I had cancer while I was struggling to do up my bra. Why couldn't he at least have waited until I was respectable? Then he didn't explain anything. Just told me to go to Admissions and arrange to come in for an operation.'

Clarissa's experience was completely different. 'The surgeon asked if I minded being seen by a student. I did, but I thought I ought to say yes and the poor young man was more nervous than I was. Then the specialist examined me and left the room while I got dressed. When I came out he asked me to sit down and explained that I'd got a small cancer and could have just the lump removed. He told me to take my time and asked if I would I like a cup of tea. My partner, Jim, had offered to come to the hospital with me, but I didn't want him to have to take time off work. How I wished I had let him come! They sent me off to see the breast-care nurse and she arranged everything – even offering to get someone to take me home.'

Further tests

These tests are explained in more detail in Chapter 6.

Mammography

Depending on what the surgeon finds in his examination, he may want you to have a mammogram, even if you've had one already. If possible, this is done during that clinic so you don't have to come back. If he is almost sure there is nothing to worry about, you may have to wait a day or two for an appointment so that the urgent mammograms can be done that day.

Ultrasound

Mammography does not show up breast changes as well in younger, premenopausal women as it does in older women, whose breasts consist mainly of fat (see Chapter 1). Younger women are more likely to sent for an ultrasound scan (see Chapter 6), which may be carried out at once or in a day or two, requiring a return visit.

Fine needle aspirates (FNAs)

The surgeon may want to remove some cells from the lump in your breast by FNA (see Chapter 6). Some people find this almost painless, no more than a little prick; but it can be more painful, like when someone not too experienced takes blood. In specialist breast clinics, a cytopathologist (see below) may be available to look at the slides immediately and you will be told the result straight away. In some clinics this is not possible, and you may have to come back in a few days for the result.

Quite the worst part for me was worrying that I would make a fool of myself. My cancer was one of the few which are tender and having a needle stuck into it was quite painful, though bearable. Other women find that an FNA of their cancer hardly hurts at all.

If you have a cyst and fluid is drawn off, that may be all that is required. If some blood is present, you may have to wait a few days for a report until the fluid has been examined under the microscope. The chances of there being an underlying cancer in a cyst are very small.

Biopsy

At your first examination, the surgeon may be able to tell you straight away what treatment you will need, or he may need to take a biopsy (a small piece of the lump) under local or general anaesthetic (see Chapter 6). If the lump turns out to be cancer, he then discusses with you the type of operation he recommends. It is up to you to put your point of view. If you wish, ask for a few days to think about it. A small delay won't do you any harm.

Chest X-ray and blood count

If you need an operation for cancer, the surgeon will probably arrange for you to have a chest X-ray and full blood count to be sure you are not anaemic. He may also decide to order a bone or liver scan (see Chapter 6).

Arranging your operation

If the surgeon can suggest a date for you to come in, you will be sent to the Admissions Office from the clinic. You will be told where to go on the day you come in, usually the day before the operation. Alternatively you may have to go home and wait for a bed to become available. If it is cancer, you won't be kept waiting long.

The bad news interview

Women can remember word for word the way in which they were told they had cancer.

It's a bit like labour. I can remember every detail of the birth of all four of my children, even though the eldest was born in 1960 and the 'baby' in 1967 – and exactly how it felt sitting in the car waiting, just be sure that it wasn't a false alarm, so that my second son was nearly born in the car park! Women go over and over in their minds what was said, and it colours everything they feel about their breast cancer and its treatment.

Some are invited to sit down, have a cup of tea and see the breast-care nurse who makes sure someone can take them home if necessary. Others are given the bald facts. They feel they are being treated like ignorant schoolgirls and left to take themselves home as best they can.

Attempts are being made to teach young medical students the

importance of the psychological aspects of physical disease, but there is a long way to go. Doctors in this country are still too patronising – I even catch myself at it, pontificating about this or that. And I am afraid we don't all give exactly the same advice, even when we're members of the same team. Doctors in any Firm (see below) have regular update meetings, but if you ask two different doctors how long it will be before your scar heals, for example, you may get two different answers – which can be very unnerving. Ask to see the consultant and get anything that is important to you sorted out with him.

Who's who at the hospital

If you have no previous experience of hospitals, it can be very confusing trying to work out who does what, who is a doctor, and who isn't.

What do you call everyone?

There are two main types of specialist doctors: physicians and surgeons. Physicians, who treat patients with medicines and radiotherapy, or report on a variety of tests (for example radiologists, pathologists and so on), and who do not perform operations, are called Doctor (Dr). In the UK surgeons, who do carry out operations, are called Mr, Ms or Mrs. They are the modern-day descendants of the barber-surgeons who were not medically trained and who looked upon physicians, who had to be present when they operated, as quacks. The custom of calling them 'Mr' rather than 'Doctor' comes from that time. For the same reason, dental surgeons in the UK are not addressed as 'Doctor'. In the USA, on the other hand, all medically qualified people are called 'Doctor', including dentists.

The Firm

The team of doctors in any speciality is called a Firm. At the top is the consultant, then the senior and junior registrars, then the house doctor and finally the students. When you see a procession marching down a corridor with a senior doctor at the front and a gaggle of students trailing at the back, that is a Firm. Medical students spend weeks or months in small groups with the various medical, surgical and obstetric Firms.

Consultants, registrars and housemen

All specialists are called consultants. If a consultant is employed by a university, he is probably also a senior lecturer or even a professor. TV soaps have made us familiar with the poor, overworked house doctor who is newly qualified and takes orders from everyone. He or she sees you daily and is your first point of contact with the Firm.

In between are the registrars. The senior registrar is a fully trained, highly qualified doctor whose next job will be as a consultant; he may well carry out your operation. Junior registrars are the next grade down. They have higher qualifications than their first medical degree, or may be taking more advanced exams. Sometimes there is also a senior house officer.

The surgeon

You will be seen first by a surgeon – the consultant or his registrar. He may be a general surgeon, or, increasingly, he will be a specialist in breast surgery.

The plastic surgeon

Surgery carried out to improve the way we look is called cosmetic or plastic surgery. If you decide to have breast reconstruction (Chapter 10), your breast surgeon may call in a plastic surgeon to perform the operation immediately your breast is removed, while you are still unconscious. If you decide to have reconstruction later, he will probably send you to a plastic surgeon. Because it is considered non-urgent under the NHS, you may unfortunately have to wait a long time. As the pressure builds up from women who want to have this, attitudes are changing.

The anaesthetist

The anaesthetist is the doctor who puts you to sleep and checks you are OK before, during and after the operation.

The oncologist

An oncologist is a doctor who specialises in the treatment of cancer by radiotherapy, by chemotherapy using anti-cancer drugs, or both. If the oncologist specialises in treatment by X-rays, he will be called a radiotherapist.

The radiologist

A radiologist is a doctor whose speciality is the interpretation of X-rays, ultrasound scans and a variety of other scans, like bone scans and liver scans. He does not generally treat patients, but may carry out very specialised treatments, specially those performed under X-ray guidance, like injecting anti-cancer drugs directly into the artery going to the liver.

The radiographer

A radiographer is a highly trained technician who carries out your mammogram, chest X-ray or bone scan. When the films are ready, a radiologist will report on them. If you need radiotherapy, the treatment is planned by the radiotherapist and a physicist, but carried out by a radiographer.

The pathologist

The pathologist is the doctor who examines tissue removed by the surgeon, whether small portions from biopsies or the whole operation specimen. If the tissue contains cancer, the pathologist determines its size and type, and checks under the microscope that the cancer has been completely removed. He also examines the lymph nodes from your armpit to see whether cancer has spread there.

The cytopathologist

The cytopathologist (or cytologist) is the doctor who specialises in the study of individual cells removed by FNA (see Chapter 6). He also reports on cervical smears, and cells in urine and sputum. In a well-run breast unit, a cytologist is in attendance to look at FNAs carried out in the clinic and issue an immediate report. In some clinics it is the cytologist rather than the surgeon who does FNAs.

The breast-care nurse

Every breast unit should have a breast-care nurse, though not all of them yet do. Under the stress of being told we have cancer or of coming round from surgery, it is difficult to take everything in. The breast-care nurse listens to your fears, real and imaginary, offers you a shoulder to cry on and helps sort out your personal problems. She explains in simple terms the news or advice from the specialist which you haven't been able to take in.

> People assume that if you are a doctor, you know all the answers and don't need reassurance. I had lots of questions but knew first hand just how busy and overworked my doctors were. There was nothing important enough for me to ask to see them specially, so it was a pleasant surprise to find that they had arranged for a breast-care nurse to visit me. I felt I could let my hair down in front of another woman, cry and say all the things I had been bottling up, not wanting to bother my doctors or worry my family. I owe a great debt to the breast-care nurse at my hospital. I am sure my recovery would have been much more fraught without her help and kindness. It was probably more difficult for her at first, having a consultant as a patient, but I was as worried and distressed as any other woman with cancer. I have watched her concerned and capable, talking to other patients. I don't know how she can remain so caring, when she is obviously rushed off her feet, and has her own young family to look after.

If you are at all worried about how your chest will look after the operation, ask the breast-care nurse to introduce you to a post-operative patient to show you what the scar will be like. If you are thinking about breast reconstruction, the breast-care nurse will know women who are happy to visit you and let you see the result.

Some people are worried that, in units with breast-care nurses, doctors will spend less time reassuring their patients. After all, it is usually the doctor who breaks bad news. Good cancer units are well aware of this and everyone spends as much time as they can explaining things, but NHS units are often busy and overstretched.

Students

At teaching hospitals, and sometimes at general hospitals, you may be examined by a student, or students may be present when you are examined by a doctor. Breasts don't have a sexual significance for doctors or students in a hospital environment; they are simply another part of the body like an arm, a leg or the abdomen. The doctor or student won't be embarrassed and will try to make you feel as comfortable as possible. If a student is very junior, he may be shy – but be patient with him: he may be the very person who later makes that breakthrough in breast cancer we all hope for.

You can refuse to let students sit in on your examination or to examine you. This happens more often with male medical students, but it is a great pity.

Two women at a clinic I attended refused to have a very charming, young male student come into the examination room. He told me that female students on the Firm got much more experience in examining women patients. It will be a long time before there are equal numbers of male and female consultants in the UK, so you are likely to be seen by a male consultant. They need the opportunity to learn as students how to treat their women patients with tact and sensitivity.

Physiotherapists

A physiotherapist is a non-medical person who is trained to carry out the prevention and treatment of a variety of diseases by physical methods, such as massage, exercise and heat. Usually a woman, she will come to see you after your operation to help get you moving again.

Nurses

Last, but certainly not least, are the nurses, the mainstay of any hospital. They are with patients 24 hours a day – albeit in shifts – and their vigilance can pick up minor problems before these escalate into catastrophes.

Patients always seem to ask the most difficult questions of the least formidable, most junior nurse, but these days even the ward sister – or whatever name is current in your hospital – isn't the dragon we, as young doctors, used to fear. Feel free to ask for their help and advice – though not at their most busy times. They will put you in touch with the breast-care nurse or with one of the doctors if your problem requires more specialist help. They are used to comforting weepy women. You really don't have to pretend in front of them.

At the breast clinic

While researching this book I spent some time at a breast clinic run by the surgeon who had carried out my operation. I wasn't a patient, and therefore couldn't quite get into the feelings of the women waiting there, but I did gain an insight into what it was like to be seen by a caring but very busy specialist. (All the doctors' names have been changed.)

The breast clinic was crowded. By mid-morning there were about 30 women waiting to be seen, four of whom were accompanied by husbands or partners. Those four women turned out not to have cancer, but it was good that they had someone reassure them that they had heard correctly, and really had nothing to worry about.

Mr Smith, the surgeon, and his senior registrar, saw all the new patients. The oncologist and his senior registrar saw anyone who needed chemotherapy or radiotherapy. No-one seemed to mind another doctor sitting in. When there were students present, the surgeon preferred only to have one at a time, so as not to make patients feel uncomfortable.

Although I know that most women with breast lumps have benign breast disease, I was still surprised to find that only one of the women I saw at my first clinic had cancer. All of them were desperately worried.

One-stop service

There was a cytologist, in attendance, Dr Brown, ready to look at any FNAs taken at the clinic (see Chapter 6). Most of the time, she could say immediately whether a lump was benign or malignant. If a patient needed a mammogram or ultrasound scan, it was carried out in the X-ray department during the morning. The patients may have had to wait a while for their hospital appointment, but at least they didn't have to wait yet again for their mammogram or ultrasound scan, or for the results of their FNA. Unfortunately, only a limited number of breast clinics has this one-stop service at the present time.

No-one likes sitting around waiting, and it's specially bad waiting somewhere like a breast clinic, where there are so many worried women. Some patients were in and out in minutes, but others took a long time to get to the bottom of their problem.

The diagnosis

Bra trouble

Three very worried women, young and old, complained of breast pain, not knowing that pain is an unusual symptom of primary breast cancer. One was a large woman who needed a heavier, more supportive bra. Another was a young woman who had just taken up a new sport. She hadn't realized that bumping her breasts up and down could cause persistent pain in the upper, outer part of the breast – the part which takes most of the strain. The third woman had recently started wearing an underwired bra which cut into her breasts, causing pain that didn't go away after she had removed her bra.

I was surprised (though I shouldn't have been) to find how much Mr Smith knew about bras, and how understanding he was. I think I was less sympathetic. I thought, 'Surely they should have realized what the trouble was?' Then I scolded myself: if it was *that* easy to work out the cause of their pain, those women would have done so.

I saw for myself that women with breast pain need reassurance more than anything else. Their faces lifted when Mr Smith told them they didn't have cancer at all, and in a kind, sympathetic fashion explained how best to deal with their problems.

Benign breast disease

Two women at the clinic had previously had cysts in their breasts. Mr Smith examined the breasts of the first woman, could feel nothing but ordered mammograms just to be absolutely sure. The mammograms showed some tiny cysts, too small to feel. She was embarrassed that she had apparently come to the clinic for nothing. Mr Smith explained the mammograms, telling her that such cysts sometimes fill up and get quite large, but then go away – a fairly common occurrence.

The other woman had a new breast lump and was very worried that this time it was cancer. Mr Smith inserted a fine needle into the cyst cavity. He drew off the fluid and then felt the place where the lump had been to make sure it had now disappeared. He warned her that she might have further cysts because she was on HRT. Women on HRT go on experiencing the features of fibrocystic change (see Chapter 2), but are advised always to take a breast lump seriously.

Doctors prefer to see patients without serious disease and with nothing to worry about, rather than miss a possible cancer.

'Nothing would make me happier', Mr Smith said, 'than to go through a whole breast clinic and find no cancers at all.'

Cancer

One elderly woman had cancer in a gland in her armpit. She'd had a breast lump removed some years before, but, because of illness, had not completed her course of radiotherapy. Mr Smith drew off some cells by FNA, and we looked at them under the microscope with Dr Brown. They were undoubtedly malignant. Mr Smith broke the news gently and sympathetically. For a moment she was going to cry, but then pulled herself together. Her daughter had more trouble holding back her tears.

'It's not so bad,' Mr Smith said. 'You'll only need to come in for a few days for me to remove the involved glands.'

The future wasn't bright but she couldn't have been dealt with in a more caring fashion.

Questions to ask

It is always worth writing down any questions you want to ask the doctor. The first time you go to hospital, you may not know you have cancer and may come unprepared. If you can, take someone with you. When you are stressed it is very difficult to take in what is said to you. Women often complain that they are not informed sufficiently about the diagnosis, treatment or possible complications – but consultants also complain that they really have explained it all.

At the clinics I sat in on, I was most impressed by the time the consultants and their registrars spent listening and explaining. Quite often, patients have hardly taken anything in, while their companions have understood it all. We all know the feeling: 'What did he say?'; 'Did he really say it was benign?' It is perfectly OK to take notes. Few people are capable of remembering more than two facts from a consultation, so it's not surprising that women can't recall exactly what was said.

You have every right to ask questions and find out as much as possible. In this country, we almost feel embarrassed to question doctors, as if we were questioning their skill by daring to ask. Don't feel that way; ask about whatever is troubling you. Several studies show that women have fewer psychological problems if they understand what is being done and why.

Questions you may wish to ask before surgery

- Is it cancer?
- Has it spread?
- How long will I be in hospital?
- Can I have just the lump removed or will I need a mastectomy?
- Will breast reconstruction be possible?
- When will I be able to have breast reconstruction?
- Will I need to have radiotherapy and/or chemotherapy afterwards?

Questions you may wish to ask before radiotherapy or chemotherapy

- Do I really need it?
- How many visits will be required?
- Will my hair fall out? If it does can I get a wig?
- Will I feel bad?
- I have booked a holiday. Can it be fitted in?

Questions you may wish to ask when your treatment is finished

- Is there anything I shouldn't do?
- Can I do everything at home?
- Is it OK to have sex?
- Can I have another baby?
- When can I go back to work?
- Will it recur?

8

Surgery for breast cancer

At your first appointment (see Chapter 7), you may be seen, and later treated, by a surgeon who is a specialist in the treatment of breast disease, or by a general surgeon. The Government plan is that Cancer Units, staffed by a team of experts, will be set up in district hospitals for the treatment of common cancers like breast, lung, stomach and bowel cancer. There will be about 200 units, each seeing 100–150 patients a year and serving a population of 200,000–300,000. In addition, there will be Cancer Centres where most radiotherapy will be given, and where rarer cancers will be treated, as well as the more common ones. Most Cancer Centres will be part of a large general hospital.

The variation in the number of deaths from breast cancer between different areas of the country has been much publicized. The establishment of dedicated Cancer Units, available to women wherever they live, should improve the standard of care throughout the country. There are small units which have offered excellent treatment in the past, but now it is recommended that all breast surgery should be carried out by experienced breast surgeons who treat at least 50 cases a year. In fact, both lumpectomy and mastectomy are fairly straightforward operations. It is not the actual operation that is crucial, except to your appearance – though perhaps the importance of a good-looking result should be as much emphasized in this country as it is in the USA. What makes the difference is treatment by an expert *team* of surgeons, oncologists and breast-care nurses, all of whom specialize in breast cancer.

Removal of your primary breast cancer is most often the first line of treatment. However, if your cancer is large, it may need first to be treated with radiotherapy or chemotherapy, or you may not be well enough to have surgery and need to be treated medically (see Chapter 9). Even if the cancer has spread elsewhere in the body, it is often best to remove the cancer in the breast itself to prevent ulceration (breaking through the skin).

The two types of surgery carried out for breast cancer are *lumpectomy* (removal just of the cancer), and *mastectomy* (removal of the whole breast, from the Greek words *mastos* meaning 'breast', and *ektome* meaning 'cutting out').

Lumpectomy

About 50–60% of breast cancers can be removed by lumpectomy, leaving a complete but smaller breast. Most surgeons will also want to remove the lymphatic glands in the armpit of the affected side to check whether cancer cells have spread there.

There is a greater risk of recurrence in the remaining breast if you have a lumpectomy rather than a mastectomy, so most women have radiotherapy after a lumpectomy. This aims to kill off any cancer cells which might remain in the breast tissue left behind. If you do have a recurrence, you can have a mastectomy later. It is very disappointing, but does not adversely affect how long you live.

Quadrantectomy is removal of a quadrant (a whole segment) of the breast for larger cancers. It is likely to leave a larger hollow in the breast, which may need reconstruction or a breast-form (see Chapter 10) to improve its appearance.

If the cancer is very tiny, too small for the surgeon to feel, he may need to insert a very fine wire, guided by X-rays, into the area where the cancer was found on the mammogram. The cancer is then removed, including the wire, and the lump is X-rayed to make sure the small cancer was taken out.

Because CIS (carcinoma *in situ* – see Chapter 4) is often widespread in the breast, in the past women with CIS were recommended mastectomy. The present view is that lumpectomy (removal only of the lump) is all that is required, provided that the CIS is localized in one area of the breast, and that when it is removed, the edges are seen under the microscope to be clear of tumour. The prognosis of CIS is excellent, with a five-year survival of over 98%. This means that a tiny proportion (less than 2%) of patients with CIS must have had areas of invasive cancer not seen under the microscope. Trials are under way to see whether radiotherapy or Tamoxifen will help to prevent recurrence or spread.

It may not be possible to breast-feed after lumpectomy if it is followed by radiotherapy, but even after mastectomy nature makes up for the loss of one breast by producing more milk on the other side.

Mastectomy

Mastectomy is removal of the whole breast. There are four kinds:

1 Simple mastectomy. This involves the removal of the breast, together with an ellipse (a pointed oval) of skin including the nipple. All or some of the lymph nodes in the armpit are usually also removed.

2 Modified radical mastectomy. This comprises simple mastectomy, plus the removal of the small pectoralis muscle which makes the complete removal of the lymph glands in the armpit easier. Though this is a larger operation than simple mastectomy, the scar it leaves is similar.

3 Subcutaneous mastectomy. In this operation, the breast mound is removed but the overlying skin and nipple are left behind. It was recommended for widespread CIS, but provided the area of CIS can be removed completely, it is often now treated by wide lumpectomy. Subcutaneous mastectomy is also used for women who have their breasts removed prophylactically (before cancer develops). They may want this because they come from a very high-risk cancer family, or because they have had several benign lumps removed and can't face the worry that the next one will be cancer. Since some cancer cells could possibly lurk in the remaining breast tissue under the nipple, some surgeons instead advise simple mastectomy for these women.

4 Radical mastectomy. In this operation the breast, overlying skin and nipple, underlying chest muscles and lymph glands in the armpit are removed. This type of operation should be only a historical relic. It dates from the time when it was believed that cancer spread outwards from the breast, so if you removed enough tissue you could be sure you had 'got it all out'. We now know that cells may spread to the lymph glands and distant organs very early, and that the deformity produced by radical mastectomy was without benefit.

Lymph glands in the armpit are removed (axillary clearance) so that the pathologist can determine whether cancer has spread there, and the stage your cancer has reached (see Chapter 4). This will influence the decision as to whether you need to have chemotherapy (Chapter 9).

It used to be taught that if the cancer was under the nipple, lumpectomy was not suitable. The assumption was that a breast without a nipple was not worth having, but many women would rather not lose their breast. They can always choose to have a false, stick-on nipple, or just not bother, or consider nipple reconstruction (see Chapter 10). If your cancer is large in relation to the size of your breast, lumpectomy might not leave a breast that would look good. In this case you may be advised to have a mastectomy.

Seeing a woman who has had a mastectomy

If you are advised to have a mastectomy, or you choose to have it rather than lumpectomy, ask to see someone who has already had the operation. Many of us have a picture in our minds of a deep hole where the breast has been.

Until I wrote this book, I had not actually seen the chest of someone who'd had a mastectomy. At one of the self-help groups I visited, Phoebe showed me her breast and breast-form (prosthesis). I was surprised at how 'normal' she looked. It's true, one side was flat – but the other breast was fine. When she had on her bra and prosthesis there was no way you could tell one breast was absent.

Some women, after they have had a mastectomy, have problems letting their daughters see their chests.

Julie has three teenage daughters and it was months before she allowed them to see her without clothes. 'Is that all?', Tina, the eldest, said. 'I was expecting something really terrible. I wish you'd let us see you before. I've been having nightmares about it, but it's nothing.' She hugged Julie. 'We just thank God you're OK, Mummy.'

Surgery and the menstrual cycle

Some studies have suggested that you are less likely to have a recurrence of breast cancer if surgery is carried out in the second half of your menstrual cycle. Some surgeons try to operate so as to coincide with these dates, but others have found no such difference.

Breast cancer in elderly women

Many otherwise healthy, elderly women can take surgery and radio-therapy in their stride. They are often as concerned about avoiding mastectomy as younger women, and may have many years of life remaining. In the UK the average expectation of life for women is 80 (74 for men). Figures also show that if a woman lives to be 60 she can expect to live to 83; if she lives to 80, the expectation of life becomes 89. The longer you live, the greater the age you can expect to live to – because you have avoided or got over the diseases which have carried off younger people.

Mastectomy in men

In men, appearance is less important and mastectomy more often performed. Because male breasts are smaller, a graft may occasionally be required to make good the gap in the skin after the cancer is removed.

Lumpectomy or mastectomy?

It is your breast. If the surgeon recommends one operation and you would rather have another, you can ask for a second opinion. The next surgeon may advise the same, but at least you will feel you've talked the subject through. You don't have to make an immediate decision. A few days' delay, or even a couple of weeks, won't affect your chances of cure. It is the months and years women put off going to see the doctor that are bad. If you have a choice, take your time deciding. Often your immediate reaction is to want the cancer out at any cost. If you have a little time to reflect, you may decide you would prefer a lumpectomy. Up to 30% of women who are offered the choice opt for mastectomy. They would prefer to feel that their tumour is all out and not come back to hospital for four to six weeks of radiotherapy.

> Jane was offered lumpectomy. ' "No," I told the doctor', she said. ' "It makes me ill just thinking about hospitals. I want my cancer out and finished. I'm not coming back week after week for X-ray treatment." My old fellow told me to do whatever I thought best.'

However, depending on what the cancer looks like under the microscope, and whether there is cancer in the lymph glands (the grade and stage of the tumour – see Chapter 4), some patients who have had a mastectomy still need radiotherapy afterwards.

The operation

Going into hospital

Take a loose night-dress or some pyjamas which button down the front to make examination and nursing-care easier. You will need a pair of slippers for going to the bathroom, and a bedjacket or cardigan. You spend a lot of time sitting up in bed. It is less embarrassing to be seen by a lot of strangers in a bed-jacket than in a nightie, and in the winter hospitals can be a bit draughty. If you don't have a night-dress or pyjamas, the hospital can lend you some.

Pack your toilet bag, and include your make-up if it makes you feel better. It can get very boring in hospital, especially if you are used to being active, so take some books or magazines. You will need a phone-card or change for telephone calls and for newspapers. It's best not to take valuables to hospital with you. Give anything precious to the ward sister for safe-keeping.

Before the operation

If you are in a teaching hospital, a medical student may come and 'clerk' you. This means taking a full medical history. He or she asks you what illnesses you have had, how you found out you had cancer, and so on – and then examines you thoroughly. If the student is male, you can ask to have a woman student instead – though it is hard on male students, who therefore get less experience.

A qualified junior doctor (house surgeon) who is part of the surgical team, checks you over. He asks you to sign the consent form in which you agree to have your operation. It is unusual these days for surgeons not to have decided before they start whether they are going to do a lumpectomy or a mastectomy. Sometimes, though, it may have been difficult to decide before surgery whether your lump is cancer or not. You may therefore be asked to sign for either operation, depending on what the surgeon and pathologist find when the lump is removed. If you feel strongly, say so. You can write 'Not mastectomy' on the consent form if you are worried. The surgeon can sew up the wound, discuss what to do next with you when you have got over the anaesthetic, and carry out a mastectomy in a few days if it is needed.

The anaesthetist comes to see you to check that you are fit for surgery and order your pre-medication – the drugs that are given an hour or so before your operation to make you drowsy. You may not be quite asleep when you are wheeled to the side-room off the operating theatre – the anaesthetics room. There you will be put soundly asleep before you are taken into the operating theatre.

Discussing side-effects

The media often highlight people who weren't warned about the possible side-effects of surgery, but it is difficult to strike a happy medium between scaring patients half to death and keeping important information from them. Your surgeon or your oncologist will warn you about the common complications and side-effects, though you may be one of the lucky women who has none at all.

After the operation

It is often hard to get your bearings when you come round after an anaesthetic. What I remember most about coming round was being certain that I hadn't yet had my operation. Many have the same experience.

Anaesthetics are so good these days that most people don't feel sick afterwards. If you do feel sick, tell the nurse and you will be given something take away the feeling of nausea.

If you have had a cancer removed, you will have one or two plastic drains (thin, flexible tubes) coming out of the wound. These drain any blood or fluid into a plastic bag. You will be encouraged to move around the ward as soon as possible. You feel silly to begin with, but soon get used to walking around holding the bag.

You may have a number of strange feelings in or around the operation site. They may begin when you first wake up after your operation or they may develop after some time. You may have numbness or pins and needles around the wound and along the inner side of your upper arm. Some women have an aching feeling in their wound or shoulder, which spreads down their arm. If you have had a mastectomy, you may have the sensation that your breast is still there. Some of these feelings will have gone by the time you leave hospital but some may continue for a long time.

> Sophie said she'd been treated very well at her local hospital but wished she had been told she might have pain going down her arm. She thought the operation had permanently damaged her nerves and that she'd be left with the pain for the rest of her life. It cleared up in a couple of weeks, but she would have liked to have been warned beforehand.
>
> I went on having odd pains in the side on which I'd had my operation. They were never severe enough to need even aspirins, but they niggled me. Then one day, after about three years, I realised they had gone, except for the occasional twinge.

Exercises

Your shoulder and arm may be stiff and difficult to move at first. A physiotherapist or the breast-care nurse will visit you to help get you moving and start you on gentle exercises. Take it easy and don't overdo things. If you are not offered exercises, ask the ward sister. By the time you go home, you should be able to brush your hair and do up the back of your clothes.

Going home

If you have drainage tubes in place they will be removed and you will be discharged after about five days; some women go home earlier, with drains still in position. Following removal of the tubes, fluid may collect under your skin for the first couple of weeks, and you may have some swelling and discomfort, particularly in the armpit. This is common and does not mean that there is anything to worry about. Your doctor may need to remove the fluid with a very fine needle. This is not painful, just a pinprick. Your stitches will be removed between one and two weeks after your surgery, either at the hospital clinic or by your GP. There may be slight oozing for a few days after the stitches come out. If this occurs, put a clean, dry dressing over the wound and change it every day. Any bruising will gradually fade.

When you go home you may bathe normally, unless you have been told otherwise.

The wound may be red, puckered and lumpy at first but it will flatten out with time till only a white line is visible. When it has healed soundly, you can soften it by rubbing in a non-allergenic moisturising cream once or twice a day. It is quite frightening going home with an incompletely healed scar but you will be surprised how quickly it settles down. If you are worried at any time about the condition of the wound, contact your GP or the hospital. A summary of your treatment will be sent to your GP shortly after you leave hospital.

Most mastectomy scars will be where your breast crease was, and well hidden by a bra. Surgeons try to make sure lumpectomy scars will also be hidden.

Bras and prostheses

If you have had a mastectomy you will probably be offered a temporary Cumfie breast-form designed by Betty Westgate, the founder of Breast Cancer Care (BCC – see Useful addresses). These are machine-washable and are filled with acrylic fibre which can be added or removed until it matches the other breast. When the scar has healed, you can make an appointment to be fitted for a permanent breast-form through your hospital. If you prefer, you can go direct to the BCC who have all sizes and types (see Chapter 10) and can advise you on which to get your hospital to order for you. If your breast and nipple remain tender, you may want to change to a softer bra or even wear none at all for a while.

> I bought a couple of cotton crop tops, the kind with broad shoulders, a scoop neck and very little support. The skin on my side and my nipple were very sensitive for a long time, so for nearly a year I gave up wearing bras altogether. A larger woman, however, might find this uncomfortable and need to find a bra that gives enough support while not cutting into the tender side.

Exercising your arm

Initially your arm on the operation side may be painful and stiff. It is important that you continue to do your exercises. It's OK to do gentle housework, like hanging clothes on the line, dusting, sweeping, or light gardening. Always wear gloves to protect your hands against cuts or scratches. Take it gently. You may get tired more easily that you expect. Don't lift heavy bags of shopping or suitcases for the first few weeks, and certainly not until the wound is well-healed and you have full movement of the arm and shoulder on that side. You can start driving again when you feel up to it and are able to move your arm freely and without pain.

Follow-up

You will be given appointments at the breast clinic after your operation or after radiotherapy, to check all is well. Usually it will be every three months for the first year, every six months the next year and then at least once a year for five years, and sometimes for life. Write down any questions you think of before your next appointment, and remember to ask them when you see the doctor. If you are worried at all before your next appointment – for example, if you find another lump, or anything of concern – don't wait. Ring up straight away for an earlier appointment.

Further medical treatment

Most women need some further treatment after surgery (see Chapter 9). The commonest is radiotherapy. Some will need a course of chemo-therapy. Most postmenopausal women will be prescribed Tamoxifen tablets for at least two years. Studies are under way to determine how long they should be taken after that.

If you are prescribed hormone replacement therapy (HRT) implants or vaginal creams for menopausal symptoms, you should discuss this with the doctors in the breast clinic before starting such treatment. Views differ as to whether or not HRT is wise after breast cancer.

Snacking – a word of warning

If you have been very busy before going into hospital and have time off work to recuperate, it is easy to get into the habit of snacking. You may do it for comfort, out of boredom, or just because food is so easily available at home.

> I had been a very busy person before my operation. While I was working I often went without lunch. With one thing and another, I managed to stay pretty trim. Unfortunately I didn't notice for some time after my operation that my clothes were getting tight. I had quite a lot of local discomfort after surgery and gave up wearing a bra altogether for some time. When I decided to wear a bra again, I was horrified. I could just about do it up and a big roll of fat hung over the side. Dieting and regular swimming helped but I've never really got back to my pre-operation size. My scar is perfectly OK but my waist and tummy certainly aren't!

If you have been prescribed Tamoxifen you may find it extra difficult to control your weight.

Side-effects of surgery

Lymphoedema

Lymphoedema is a condition in which a part of the body, usually the arm after breast surgery, swells and may become painful. Some of the fluid in our arms is carried back to the blood system via the lymphatic ducts which drain first into the armpit (see Chapter 1). If the ducts are blocked, fluid accumulates in the arm and makes it swell (*oedema* is Greek for 'swelling').

The lymphatic ducts may be blocked in a number of ways, for example, the removal of lymph nodes in the armpit cuts some of the ducts. After modern surgery, which is designed to produce as little damage as possible, other ducts grow out to replace those which have been damaged in the operation. In time the normal drainage is restored. In the days of radical mastectomy, many more women suffered lymphoedema – in fact, it was almost considered part of the price of getting rid of the primary cancer.

Radiotherapy to the lymph nodes in the armpit can also cause lymphoedema. The combination of surgery plus radiotherapy to the armpit is particularly likely to lead to lymphoedema, and is best avoided if possible. If cancer spreads to the lymph glands in the armpit, lymph-oedema can result. So-called benign lymphoedema is not due to cancer, but is often due to the lymphatic ducts not forming properly during development.

It is not unusual to have some swelling of your breast or arm after surgery to your armpit, but the swelling usually goes away in a few days. Many women have a little lymphoedema in crease marks or over the muscle of their shoulder, that does not get any worse. If the fluid is allowed to remain in the arm, it acts as an irritant. Scar-tissue, in which new ducts cannot form, is laid down and the swelling becomes permanent. It is therefore important to deal with any swelling as soon as possible.

Sometimes lymphoedema occurs some time after surgery. It may be set off by insect bites or infected scratches, so you should always be careful of your arm on the operated side. It is also one of the less frequent ways in which breast cancer can first show itself. If it occurs some time after your operation without being caused by something obvious like an infected cut or insect bite, go and see your doctor just to be sure.

Treatment of lymphoedema

Report any swelling in your hand or arm to your doctor at once, as it is much more easily dealt with at an early stage by gentle massage and compression bandaging. You may need to wear an elasticated stocking on your arm, particularly at night, and it will help if you sleep with your arm propped up on a pillow. You may need to wear a stocking during the day in hot weather, when your arm swells more. At the present time only pink stockings are available but if you have a black skin you can dye the stocking very successfully with fabric dye.

> Tony said it made a lot of difference to her confidence when she dyed her arm stocking dark brown. The bright pink against her dark skin made her feel self-conscious. She was also one of the first black women to be fitted with a black breast-form (see Chapter 10).

The gentle mobilizing exercises you were prescribed after surgery are also helpful for lymphoedema. Manual Lymph Drainage is a special massage technique which helps to remove the fluid. If there is a lymphoedema clinic at your hospital someone there may be skilled in this method. If not, contact the Lymphoedema Support Network (see Useful addresses). If you have a willing partner or friend, they can learn the techniques of compression bandaging and massage.

It is not usually possible to operate to remove the swelling, because the fluid re-forms. How much you drink, or whether or not you take anti-diuretics, does not affect lymphoedema.

Taking care

You need to take great care of your arm if you have lymphoedema. Wear thick gloves when you do anything which might damage your fingers, such as washing up or gardening – or avoid them. Remove underarm hair with a depilatory cream or an electric razor. Any infection should be taken seriously. If you cut yourself, clean and wash the area thoroughly and apply an antiseptic. Insect bites can cause a nasty reaction, so if you go out in the evening in an area where you might get bitten use an insect repellent. If you do get bitten or if there is redness, swelling or tenderness round a cut or scratch, go to your doctor immediately. It is best to keep your arm out of the sun, but if you are on holiday and cannot easily avoid the sun while walking around, use a high-factor non-allergenic sun-cream on your arm. Always offer the unaffected arm if you need to have an injection, or a blood sample or your blood pressure taken. Normal exercise is good for your arm, but don't carry heavy shopping with that arm, or use it for vigorous pulling or pushing.

Don't wear clothes which are tight around the armhole: they make the swelling worse. Armholes which are too tight can be dealt with by unpicking the sleeve and cutting the armhole larger. New sleeves can be made out of a matching or contrasting fabric and the spare fabric used for a belt or bandeau – or one more duster. When shopping, look for clothes with wide armholes and investigate maternity clothes which are often cut loosely around the upper arm. These days they can be very fashionable, and look good worn with a belt.

Areas of numbness and odd pains

Many women have areas of numbness over the breast, down their arm or on the back of the side operated on following surgery for breast cancer. These may be quite tiny or cover areas as big as your hand. You may have pins and needles or stabbing pains especially just after your operation. These usually get better with time, but the areas of numbness may remain.

I don't often think about the numb area I have on my back and near the scar on my breast. It's only when I have a feel before my regular check-up to make sure I can't detect a recurrence that I am aware that the numbness is still there. The odd pains took several years to finally disappear though even after five years I still get occasional twinges.

9

Medical treatment of breast cancer

Treatment after surgery

Medical (that is non-surgical) treatment of cancer – whether radiotherapy, chemotherapy or hormone therapy, or any combination of these – is usually given after surgery. It is designed to kill off any cancer cells remaining in the breast elsewhere after the tumour has been removed, and to prevent recurrence. Doctors call this 'adjuvant therapy' (from the Latin *adjuvare* to help). Your treatment will be individually planned by the breast cancer team and will depend on a number of factors including the pathologist's report, whether you are pre- or postmenopausal, and whether the cancer has spread. If these treatments are given before surgery they are called 'neo-adjuvant therapy'. Treatment given to improve the quality of life in cases of advanced cancer, or to deal with symptoms like bone pain, is called 'palliative therapy' (see Chapter 14).

A word of warning. Doctors call all medicines drugs. If they ask you what drugs you are taking, they mean medicines. They are not implying that you use illegal substances.

Radiotherapy

Radiotherapy is treatment by X-rays. This may be given externally, in a similar way to a diagnostic chest X-ray but with a much more powerful machine, or internally from radioactive wires implanted around the tumour. Radiotherapy is recommended for all patients after lumpectomy and for some, depending on the stage and grade of their tumour (see Chapter 4), after mastectomy too. Its role is to prevent local recurrence; it does not influence survival.

These days radiotherapy facilities are concentrated at fewer centres mainly for reasons of economy so you may find you have to travel to another hospital for your treatment. Some women will be eligible to have their fares paid (see Chapter 13).

External radiotherapy

Actively growing cells like cancer cells are very sensitive to X-rays. Because normal cells are also affected to some extent, radiotherapists take great care to focus the beam of X-rays accurately and to shield normal tissues. When your treatment is being worked out, a minute spot of ink is inserted under your skin to form a tiny tattoo. This enables the radiographers to focus the beam on exactly the right place each time. Your first appointment is called a 'simulation session', because it is used to decide on your position for the forthcoming treatments and simulates (is like) the real thing. Your feet will rest against blocks and your hand will be placed to grip a bar above your head. You will have test X-rays to be sure the beam covers your breast.

To maximise the damage to cancer cells and minimise the damage to normal cells, treatment is given in fractions (several small doses). Normal cells are able to recover more quickly from these small amounts of radiation than are cancer cells. External radiotherapy for breast cancer is usually given daily on an out-patient basis, from Monday to Friday, with a rest over the weekend. Treatments are carried out for four to six weeks. Your consultant is unlikely to agree to an interruption or shortening of the course to enable you to go on holiday.

> We had arranged to meet our daughter in Barcelona when my course of radiotherapy was finished, but I got the dates wrong and wanted to miss the last session. My doctor said, 'No way', and I was able to change the flight. It cost a bit more but neither the oncologist nor I would have forgiven ourselves if I had had an early recurrence. We'd both have felt it was our fault. Looking back five years later I feel a bit guilty for even asking.

Lots of women plan to escape on holiday immediately after their last treatment, but discuss this with the consultant. Remember that X-ray machines can break down or need servicing. Ask him what would be a sensible gap to leave, just in case, when booking your holiday.

Each treatment takes only a few minutes and it is unusual to feel any immediate effects – though many women get more tired as the course of treatments go on.

> When I had cancer, I had my radiotherapy first thing in the morning and then went up to my department to carry out a full day's work. I hadn't really believed that irradiating such a small proportion of my body would affect me. To begin with I felt fine, but during the month's course of treatment I was surprised to find how tired I got. In retrospect, I think it would have been better to take some time off. People vary very much in their response to radiotherapy. The woman whose treatment was just after mine had no ill effects at all.

With external radiotherapy you do not become radioactive in any way, your hair does not fall out (except any hair in the path of the beam, like in the armpit and around the nipple), and you can lead a normal life, receiving visitors, hugging and kissing children and grandchildren.

The loneliness of radiotherapy

The benefit of killing cancer cells outweighs any possible ill effects, but it is important that the radiographers who work with X-rays all day long, are not exposed. They will explain that you will be left alone in the treatment room for the few minutes the beam is on, but that they will be watching you by remote TV and that they can hear you. If you are worried about being left alone with a large machine looming over you, talk to them about it and they will reassure you.

When radiotherapy finishes

After coming in every day for their radiotherapy and feeling that help is readily at hand, some women feel cut off and very much on their own when their course of treatment is finished. The breast-care nurse can tell you if there is a self-help group at your hospital. Alternatively, phone one of the cancer charities which keeps a list of self help groups and counsellors (see Useful addresses).

Large breast cancers

If your cancer is large, the doctors may recommend that, before surgery, it is treated by radiotherapy and chemotherapy or by one or other of these, to kill the cancer cells. In many cases the tumour will shrink enough for it to be removed by lumpectomy rather than mastectomy, but specialists cannot yet be sure whether surgery can be avoided altogether after this treatment. They may not be able to feel the lump any more, and it may not show on a mammogram. There is, however, the chance that a few cancer cells may still be lurking in the breast tissue.

Studies are being carried out to see whether treatment of smaller cancers by chemotherapy before surgery will be of benefit to the patient.

Side-effects of radiotherapy

Effects on your skin and breast

Though radiotherapy is designed to affect normal tissues as little as possible, the scar and the overlying skin of your chest on the operated side may become itchy, red or tender. Some women find their breast feels or looks swollen and becomes painful. You will be told not to use perfumes, deodorants or anything on that side which might irritate the skin. Some hospitals recommend that you don't wash that side during treatment, while others suggest you just splash yourself with water and pat yourself dry gently without rubbing. If your skin does get sore, you should keep water off the treatment area completely and mention it to the hospital on your next visit. You will probably be prescribed a mild, soothing cream.

> Janet told me that not being able to wash that side ruined the holiday she went on just after her treatment finished. She was still depressed from the news that she had cancer, and was tired after radiotherapy. She was sure she smelled awful, especially as it was hot. 'I was so ratty,' she said 'I spoilt the holiday for my husband and children.'

She needn't have worried. The glancing X-rays which reach the skin of the armpit dry up the sweat glands.

> I didn't start sweating or regrow hair in my armpit for some years after radiotherapy, and even now the hair is very sparse on that side. This is an advantage in that you don't have to shave on that side for a long time.

The area irradiated often remains slightly darker than the skin on the other side, especially if you have dark skin. You will be advised not to expose the irradiated area to sun for up to two years, and then only after applying a high factor sun block.

General effects

Some women have no side-effects at all; others find that radiotherapy makes them feel tired or weak, but this often takes time to come on. Some women go on feeling tired for some months afterwards. Occasionally women develop anorexia (go off their food) or feel sick, but this is unusual. Eating small tasty meals can help, and there are very effective drugs to treat nausea.

It does not make the hair fall out, apart from the hair in your armpit on that side. It does not cause infertility, or an early menopause, unless directed at the ovaries.

Radiotherapy departments try to arrange things so that you don't sit around waiting with lots of seriously ill patients. If you do, it can be depressing. Find the sister in radiotherapy or the breast-care nurse and talk it through. We are grown-ups and have to face unpleasant things sometimes. Seeing other patients worse off may make you feel how lucky you are by comparison.

Effects on other tissues

You may have pins and needles or shooting pains in the shoulder or arm, but these can occur after surgery alone (see Chapter 8). These pains can be treated with a mild painkiller and generally they go away with time. In the days when much higher doses of X-rays were given, some women suffered scarring in their lungs or heart, or damage to the nerves that cross the armpit, and developed distressing weakness and pain. The armpit is now, therefore, irradiated with great care to avoid this. If you are one of the women who have experienced this problem, you can contact a self-help group called RAGE (Radiotherapy Action Group Exposure – see Useful addresses).

No treatment is entirely without risk, but with modern radiotherapy this is minimal.

Internal radiotherapy

For internal (interstitial) radiotherapy the patient is given a general anaesthetic, fine tubes are placed around and under the cancer or the site from which it was removed. They are then loaded with radio-active wires (at present usually iridium-192). In some countries, such as France, it may be given as the only treatment for breast cancer. In the UK, however, it is generally felt that the scarring and skin reaction produced by the amount of radiation required may cause more damage than the surgical removal of the tumour. A few centres in the UK use internal irradiation, usually to 'sterilise' the tumour site after the tumour has been removed.

As the wires are radioactive you are nursed in a single room in hospital and you cannot be visited by children or pregnant women. The treatment takes three to six days. After, this the tubes are removed and you can see or touch whoever you like.

Chemotherapy

Chemotherapy is treatment by anti-cancer (cytotoxic) drugs which are either given as tablets, or put directly into the blood stream by means of a drip into a vein. It is prescribed for women who have cancer in their lymph nodes, and many would recommend it for all premenopausal breast cancer patients. Sometimes your oncologist wishes to use a Hickman line, a semi-permanent tube which is inserted into the large vein at the root of your neck under local anaesthetic. This tube is sometimes connected to a very small pump which dispenses the anti-cancer drugs continuously. You can go home with a Hickman line, and move about as normal. When treatment is complete, the tube is slipped out leaving a tiny scar.

As with radiotherapy, the drugs used also affect normal tissues. The aim of treatment is to selectively damage the cancer cells, which are dividing and growing more rapidly than normal cells, and are therefore more sensitive to these drugs. If your drugs are given by drip, treatment may take a few hours. You can walk around holding the infusion-stand, sit and chat and go to the loo. If you get bored sitting about, take a book to read or some letters to write. The oncologist's main concern is to treat your cancer in the most effective way. It may be possible to arrange your treatment so you feel OK for special family events, but don't count on it.

Combinations of drugs are usually used in the treatment of breast cancer, as each drug has a slightly different action. The main drugs used in treatment of breast cancer are cyclophosphamide, methotrexate and 5-fluouracil, a combination known as CMF. They are given by drip at about three-weekly intervals over a six month period. If the aim of treatment is to shrink a breast cancer which is too large for surgery, often doxorubicin (previously called Adriamycin) or other drugs are added to the cocktail.

High dose treatment over a short period

Several cancer centres around the world are testing the effect of large doses of mixtures of powerful chemotherapeutic drugs given over a short period – especially to patients whose breast cancer has spread. When used together, these drugs cause very severe damage to stem cells (cells from which blood cells are formed). Patients having this treatment must therefore have some of their stem cells removed beforehand, ready to be replaced when chemotherapy is completed. Stem cells used to be collected from the bone marrow where they are formed, but now they are harvested from the blood. Injections of a blood-growth factor are given, and when the blood cell count is high enough, blood is taken from a vein just like any blood test or donation of blood. The stem cells are concentrated and kept frozen until the course of drugs is completed, when they are thawed and re-injected into the patient.

High-dose treatment certainly causes some tumours to shrink, but until these trials are completed, we will not know whether patients will go on to live longer. This treatment has to be carried out in centres which regularly carry out bone marrow or stem cell transplants, and it is extremely expensive. Because your stem cells, including immune cells, are destroyed during treatment, there is a danger of infection and bleeding. Isolation and very careful nursing are required, and with such high doses side-effects like nausea and hair loss are more frequent.

Side-effects of chemotherapy

There has been so much publicity about the side-effects of chemotherapy that it is not surprising that many women dread it. Some women seem to suffer no side-effects, or very few. In some women the side-effects of chemotherapy wear off almost as soon as the treatment is finished. Others go on feeling under the weather for some months. Some find their memory is poor while they are on treatment, but this seems to get better with time. The side effects of radiotherapy and chemotherapy are more marked when they have to be given at the same time.

Nausea, loss of appetite and mouth soreness

Most people have heard of the nausea associated with taking cytotoxic drugs, and certainly if no precautions are taken, they do make you feel sick and may even make you vomit. People used to dread their next dose and even the smell of an antiseptic with its hospital associations was enough to make them feel ill. Nausea can be greatly reduced with adequate treatment, but women who have had chemotherapy often find its associations remain for years.

> Pamela was due for her annual check-up and met me in the canteen where she used to dawdle two years before, whenever she arrived too early for her chemotherapy. I wondered why she had brought her own sandwiches and drink. 'I know it's daft,' she said, 'but the thought of collecting food from that counter is too awful. I just can't.' She also said that though she'd been quite unwell on chemotherapy, if she had to have another course she would. 'After all,' she said, 'what's six months in a whole lifetime?'

Nowadays anti-emetics (drugs which stop you feeling and being sick) are given with the cytotoxic drugs, or even before you receive treatment. It is unusual not to be able to control this unpleasant side-effect. If you feel sick on the anti-emetic your doctor has chosen, don't try to be brave, tell him or the chemotherapy sister and they will prescribe something stronger.

Some women aren't sick but lose their appetite or get diarrhoea. Drink plenty, and eat small meals more often than usual, preferably a few hours before your treatment rather than directly afterwards. Some women find it helpful to wear the acupressure wrist bands designed to prevent sea sickness, and relaxation techniques can help you deal with feeling queasy at the thought of your next visit. Ask the chemotherapy sister or contact BACUP for a leaflet (see Useful addresses). If you have diarrhoea, reduce the amount of fruit and fibre in your diet till it gets better. If the smell of cooking upsets you, persuade someone else to do it. Mouth-washes help with soreness.

Hair-loss

Not all chemotherapy drugs cause your hair to fall out (technically called alopoecia) and even if the drug you are prescribed can cause this, not everyone is affected. The drugs most likely to cause hair-loss are called anthracyclines – the one most commonly used for breast cancer is doxorubicin (previously called Adriamycin). However, if your head is kept cool while the chemotherapy drugs are being given, the chances of hair-loss are less. If you are prescribed one of these drugs, you will probably be offered a cold cap. This is elasticated like a shower cap and is filled with ice. It is put on 15 minutes before the drugs are given and is left on for about 30–50 minutes afterwards.

Not everyone can stand a cold ice bag on their head, and some women who successfully used one to avoid hair loss feel ill just at the sight of a bag of ice-cubes.

> Sarah fainted in the large supermarket where she always shops. 'It was all those bags of ice in the freezer,' she said. 'It brought it all back, and it wasn't that bad at the time, just freezing cold, that's all.'

Have your hair cut short if possible as the weight of long hair pulls more. Comb your hair gently and use a very mild shampoo. Don't use rollers or a very hot hair drier. If your hair does fall out the best way to deal with hair in the bed is to vacuum it up or to wear a net or cap. If you are prescribed a drug which can cause hair-loss under the NHS you can have a wig made beforehand just in case. If it is ordered while you are an in-patient, it is free of charge; otherwise, unless you are on some sort of benefit, you may have to make a contribution.

> Barbara, an attractive forty-year-old banker, was just about to take up a more senior post when she discovered a lump in her breast. It was too large for immediate surgery so first she had radiotherapy and then chemotherapy. She got through radiotherapy with little in the way of side-effects, but was devastated at the possibility of losing her hair. The consultant convinced her that she really needed to have the course of treatment. So she went to the wigmaker, who, she said, was a real sweetie. She had ordered an everyday wig matching her hair on the NHS, and a vivid auburn one for evening wear – a colour she'd always wanted to try.

Some women really don't seem to mind losing their hair, and regard it as a bit of an adventure.

> Edith was pleased to have the chance of seeing what it was like as a blonde instead of mid-mouse. She said her friends recognised her neither with her wig nor with her short hair, which regrew dark and curly. Both made her feel much more attractive.

Some women are quite happy to go around at home with no hair, but feel better putting on a wig when they go out, or answer the door.

Marjorie was a 62-year-old retired teacher whose hair fell out completely. She said she only wore her wig for the sake of the family. Whenever she got hot, like when she was cooking, she took it off. She had always dyed her greying hair to please her husband, but when it grew again it was curly instead of straight. She liked it so much she refused to dye it any longer. In spite of her grey hair, she looked nowhere near her age.

Once the treatment is over, hair always regrows but it may look different. Some people find that instead of the straight hair they've had all their lives, the new growth is curly. You can expect to have a full head of hair three to six months after your treatment is finished.

Effects on the blood

Cells which are constantly replaced throughout life, like normal blood cells, are also affected by cytotoxic drugs. This may cause certain side effects. You may become:

- anaemic (short of red cells) which makes you pale and easily tired;
- leucopoenic (short of white cells) which makes you more prone to infections;
- thrombocytopoenic (short of platelets) which makes you bleed more readily.

That is why, before starting treatment and before each subsequent dose, you will have your blood tested to make sure it is safe to continue. After each cytotoxic drug treatment, the number of your red and white cell blood cells (your blood count) goes down – the lowest point is called the nadir – and then they recover. You may find you have to postpone your next treatment for a week or so for this recovery to take place. It is important that you tell your doctor immediately if you get an infection of any kind. It must be treated promptly because your immune system is not working at full strength because of the cytotoxic drugs.

Because your blood count has to be monitored sometimes your treatment will have to be put off if your blood hasn't recovered sufficiently. This can make the planning of your life during chemotherapy difficult.

Mary said 'I could never guarantee to be at work, and though everyone was most understanding I felt horrible being unreliable.'

Most employers are understanding, but it is only fair to warn them that though you may wish to carry on working, you won't always know beforehand if you will feel up to it. It is courteous to give them as much notice as possible of your time off so that they can plan too. Many women are able to continue working, but if you have a demanding job it may be best to assume you won't want to work while having chemotherapy. Your hospital doctor or GP will be happy to write to your employer if you wish him to do so. Families need to be aware that you may sometimes not be up to housework, cooking or shopping.

Contraception and infertility

Your periods may stop during chemotherapy but restart later, so you need to take adequate contraceptive measures. Up to 40% of women having chemotherapy experience an early menopause. Their periods stop completely and they stop ovulating (producing eggs). If you haven't completed your family, discuss this with your oncologist before you start treatment.

Knowing that, on top of having cancer, you also can't have children may be one more blow for you to deal with.

Immunisation before going abroad

Consult your doctor before planning a trip abroad to a country for which immunisations are required. While you are having chemotherapy you should not have any which use live viruses or bacteria: polio, measles, German measles (rubella), MMR (the triple vaccine for measles, mumps and rubella), BCG (tuberculosis) or yellow fever.

Hormone therapy

About 50% of breast cancers need the circulating sex hormones in your blood to survive and grow. Even after the menopause we continue to produce some female hormones, so if yours is a cancer that needs them, cutting off their supply may reduce the size of the cancer, or prevent it recurring.

The female sex hormones, oestrogen and progesterone, are mainly produced in the ovaries. Adrenal hormones can be converted into female sex hormones, mainly in fat (see Chapter 1). This is one explanation for the possible increased incidence of breast cancer in obese women.

Tamoxifen

Tamoxifen is the most widely-used hormone treatment of breast cancer. It was developed as an anti-fertility drug, though not used as such, and it was found in the laboratory to stop the growth of breast cancer cells. Its anti-cancer effect occurs mainly because it blocks the action of oestrogen, so those cancers that are ER-positive (see Chapters 1 and 4, and Glossary) either stop growing or get smaller. Tamoxifen also increases the production of tumour suppressing substances by the body itself, and so it has some effect on cancers which are ER-negative (that is which do not have high levels of oestrogen receptor).

Studies carried out in many countries on thousands of women taking Tamoxifen have shown that it can reduce deaths from breast cancer by up to 25%, as well as reducing the number of cancers in the other breast. Many oncologists recommend that all post-menopausal women with breast cancer should take Tamoxifen for at least two years. Elderly women who are too frail for surgery are sometimes treated by Tamoxifen alone.

Side-effects of Tamoxifen

Most of the side-effects of Tamoxifen are regarded by doctors as mainly minor. These side-effects generally subside with time, and doctors feel that the drug's beneficial actions in prolonging life outweigh the side-effects.

Most side-effects seem to be worse in younger women. They include nausea and dizziness, hot flushes and sweats, vaginal dryness, weight gain and depression. The problem of vaginal dryness can be made even worse by loss of the desire for sex (the libido). If you are feeling less of a woman after breast surgery, have severe vaginal dryness and don't fancy sex any more, relationships with your partner can be placed under enormous strain. Older women may have already become less interested in sex, and these changes make matters worse.

At the weekly breast cancer self-help group, Flora, a newcomer, said, 'And sex with George is agony'. 'I thought it was just me,' Anne said. 'We haven't been mad on sex for some time, and I thought I was all dried up and off it because I hate Jim seeing me without my nightdress on.' There was a hubbub as everyone wanted to talk about a problem none of them had felt able to broach with their doctors, nor with the breast-care nurse. Mary added, 'And it's much worse than with the change. I'm really bone dry now.'

Doctors are mainly concerned with major side-effects, those that might actually make you ill. They may not have got round to discussing sex problems or advising you to try different lubricants in turn until you find one that suits you. For those who have passed the menopause, having hot flushes yet again is a nuisance, but bearable. Younger women find them horrid – embarrassing and another sign that the drug is making them menopausal. Putting on weight is a nuisance for quite a number of women.

> Lilian was fed up about putting on weight. She had just spent a couple of years getting down to her target weight and on Tamoxifen she had put it all back on again. 'Still,' she said, 'if it's my figure or me I'll plump for plump.'

Women taking Tamoxifen have a two to three fold increase in cancer of the endometrial lining of the womb, which is about as frequent as cervical cancer. Some women have vaginal 'spotting' without having cancer or any other changes in their endometrium, but it can be very frightening. Any vaginal discharge or bleeding should be taken seriously and treated promptly. If cancer is present it can usually be adequately treated by hysterectomy alone.

A few women have had eye problems, but these mostly get better when Tamoxifen is stopped. Rare cases of liver cancer and liver damage have also been reported.

Some women have suffered from blood clots in their veins, especially if they are also on chemotherapy.

About 15% of younger, premenopausal women on Tamoxifen become menopausal. Their voice may become lower and their hair thin somewhat. If your family is not complete, you must discuss this with the oncologist.

Other hormone therapy

Progesterone

Progesterone is the hormone produced in the ovary in the second half of the menstrual cycle. It is sometimes used to treat secondary cancers which have stopped responding to Tamoxifen. It is usually given as medroxy-progesterone or as megestrol. Some women experience mild nausea, but most find that it increases their appetite and they put on weight, which can be a problem. A few have muscle cramps.

Aminoglutethamide and Lentaron

Hormones produced by the adrenal gland can be converted into female sex hormones by enzymes called aromatases. The drugs, aminoglutetha-mide and formestane (Lentaron), interfere with the action of these enzymes. They do not stop production of oestrogen by the ovaries and so are not suitable for premenopausal women. Because they also block the production of other vital adrenal hormones, women on these medicines may need tablets of cortisone, the most important adrenal hormone.

Goserelin

Goserelin (Zoladex) is a drug that acts on the part of the brain called the hypothalamus (see Chapter 1). It shuts off the releasing substances which stimulate the pituitary gland to produce gonadotrophins (hormones that stimulate the ovaries to produce oestrogen). When the pituitary does not produce gonadotrophins, the ovaries do not produce oestrogen. Goserelin is therefore a suitable drug for the treatment of breast cancer in premenopausal women, particularly if their cancers are ER-positive. Its side-effect is to produce a temporary menopause, but periods usually restart when the treatment is stopped.

Removing hormone-producing glands

Chemotherapy may itself stop the ovaries producing oestrogens by causing an early menopause. Alternatively, the production of female hormones, particularly in women before the menopause, may be stopped by surgically removing the ovaries, or by treating them with X-rays. The removal of the adrenal glands, which are a further source of oestrogens is sometimes advised, though now the drug aminoglutethamide (see above) is often given instead. None of these operations are as frequently performed as previously, now that Tamoxifen and other endocrine drugs are so widely used.

10

Breast-forms and breast reconstruction

You can restore your appearance after lumpectomy or mastectomy either with a breast-form or by having breast reconstruction. However, you don't have to have a replacement breast at all, and some women don't, especially if they are small. Others only wear their breast-form for special occasions like a job interview or an evening out. A smaller number of women feel they are making the statement that they are women, whether they have one breast or two, and don't wear a breast-form or have breast reconstruction as a matter of principle.

Breast-forms

After surgery, whether lumpectomy or mastectomy, your breast or chest wall on that side are often tender. A soft cotton bra is the most comfortable to begin with, and you will probably have been given free of charge a soft Cumfie pad to put inside your bra. You can have a permanent silicone breast-form or 'falsie' (technically called a prosthesis) free of charge under the NHS six to eight weeks after your operation, or after your radiotherapy has settled down. Although mastectomy bras are also available free of charge, most women prefer to buy a prettier bra for themselves.

After lumpectomy

If you have had a lumpectomy your breasts may still be approximately the same size, though the nipples may not be at the same level. Sometimes the operation reduces your breast by a whole size and you may need to wear a Cumfie pad to make the two sides match. This, and a small, permanent silicone breast-form, to tuck in your bra, are available free of charge.

> I discussed having breasts of two different sizes with Lorraine, an experienced assistant in a large London store. 'We can usually help customers to find a bra that will hide the difference in size,' Lorraine told me. 'Last Saturday we had a woman who hadn't had an operation and her breasts were two sizes different. We find if one manufacturer's bras don't do the trick, another's will. It just takes a bit of patience.'

If you find having one breast much larger than the other upsetting, you can discuss with your surgeon having the normal breast reduced to match. However, it won't be considered an urgent operation so you could be in for a long wait.

After mastectomy

You can have a breast-form free under the NHS, and a new one can be provided free of charge when yours shows signs of wear, if it is damaged, or if you gain or lose a lot of weight. Most breast-forms are guaranteed for one to three years depending on the type. You may find that at your hospital the fitter only comes in once or twice a week and there is only a limited range for you to choose from. If you can, make an appointment to visit the offices of BCC (Breast Cancer Care; formerly the Breast Care and Mastectomy Association of Great Britain – see Useful addresses), where they keep a large range of different types and sizes. There is a relaxed, friendly atmosphere and they have some excellent booklets. It is helpful to take along a bra you've worn previously and try to match the appearance of the other breast in that.

You can then get your hospital's appliance officer to order the prosthesis you have chosen – though it can take several weeks to get one through the hospital. If you wish, you can buy one immediately from BCC, but they are quite expensive. Ring BCC for advice if you can't get to one of their centres.

The first breast-forms were made of bags of birdseed or lentils which women put in their corsets or bras. Breast-forms are now made of hard-wearing silicone which are weighted so that they move and, under clothes, look like real breasts; they also have a small nipple 'bump' to make them look more natural.

You will be surprised at how heavy your breast-form feels at first, but you will quickly get used to it. The outer polyurethane cover is completely waterproof and unaffected by chlorine in swimming pools. To begin with breast-forms were only available tinted pink but some manufacturers are now making coloured breast-forms to match a variety of other skin types – from palest pink to dark brown. They are slightly transparent and to a large extent take on your body colour.

In hot countries you may find the polyurethane covering too sweaty for comfort, though this type is probably the most realistic looking. You can buy lighter-weight, cotton-covered breast-forms for holidays in the sun.

If you have had your operation carried out privately you will have to pay for your breast-form – though some medical insurance schemes include a contribution towards their cost and the cost of breast reconstruction. It is worth checking.

Self adhesive breast-forms

Self-adhesive breast-forms, which are held on with an adhesive pad, are available for women up to about a 36C cup. The pad has a specially formulated adhesive on one side, and a strip of Velcro on the other which attaches to a strip on the breast-form. The pads can be worn for about four to ten days, depending on how hot and sweaty you get. You can get self adhesive breast-forms under the NHS, with a box of twelve adhesive pads, but you have to pay for further supplies of pads. They can be used when swimming and would be good for holidays. However, if it is very hot the adhesive can melt.

Judy had been wearing an adhesive prosthesis for some time, but it was so hot at the seaside that it kept coming unstuck. All the other women were going topless, and being a very stout-hearted person she decided to do so too with the full support of her husband and teenage sons. 'I felt great', she said. 'I wasn't sure I had the nerve. Several women came up to congratulate me on my bravery.'

Mastectomy bras

If you want one, you can get a mastectomy bra free of charge under the NHS, but you may find you can wear your favourite bra with a prosthesis inside it. Pockets are not essential, but the NHS will fit up to two pockets a year free of charge, or you can sew tapes in an 'X' shape, behind which you slip the breast-form. The lingerie departments of large High Street stores have assistants experienced in fitting bras. If you explain the problem, they will tell you if they have someone available or will advise you where to go.

Maria, a lingerie assistant, told me that at her store there was always someone on duty who was used to dealing with women who have had surgery. 'Most women are very embarrassed the first time they come, but when they come for their next bra they treat us like old friends', she said. 'All they have to do is go into a cubicle and press the button. An experienced fitter answers the bell and they discuss your problem quietly so women in the next cubicle can't hear. We usually have at least three or four suitable bras in stock'. She showed me some sports bras suitable for smaller women as well as lacy bras suitable for women with large breasts. 'The secret is to get a well fitting bra which doesn't move and allow the breast-form to slip out over the top. If the bra is properly fitted, there is no need for a pocket.'

Marks and Spencer and Bhs (British Home Stores) have several types of suitable bras, once you know the sort of thing you are looking for. The refurbished Bhs stores have changing rooms with doors that shut for privacy, and their assistants are issued with information on bras suitable for mastectomy patients. The changing facilities in Marks and Spencer stores are behind curtains and less private, though there too you can discuss your bra discreetly with an experienced assistant.

Nightdresses, swimwear and evening wear

If you feel uncomfortable without your breast-form, you can sew a pocket into the front of your nightdress, or buy one designed for post-mastectomy women from one of the stockists on the BCC list (see Useful addresses). If you wear a nightdress with a high yoke and lace frill, you may find there is no need to bother.

Swimming is excellent exercise once your scar is properly healed. If you had radiotherapy you will be advised to keep the treated area out of the sun for up to two years, and then to use a high factor sun-block. You can adapt a swimsuit or bikini by sewing in a pocket for your breast-form, or you can buy one with preformed cups and add a bigger pad to one side. Swimsuits specially designed for post-mastectomy women can be obtained from one of the specialist suppliers on the BCC list but they are more expensive than swimsuits from your local store. Your permanent breast-form is heavy, and swimming costumes don't give the same support as a bra. It's therefore best to use a soft, Cumfie pad for swimming or cut one out of sponge. When you come out of the water just push your upper arm against the breast-form to squeeze out the water. It will dry in a very short time.

If you want to wear a low-cut evening dress, deep, strapless bras are suitable for larger women, while women with smaller breasts usually find a fairly narrow bra is quite supportive enough. If you want to wear your ordinary bra, you can get special 'converti-straps' (from BCC) which pull the back down to allow you to wear a deeply cut dress. It is better not to wear your normal breast-form as it would be too heavy for so little support, though self adhesive ones are fine. You will probably find it better to use your Cumfie.

One of my most pleasant visits was to a post-mastectomy fashion show, in which four women who'd had either one or both breasts removed were modelling clothes. They modelled everything from underwear and swimwear to everyday clothes and evening dresses. There was no way you could tell who had had breast reconstruction and who was wearing a breast-form. I overheard them swapping stories about gardening. Apparently all the bending and straightening is the best thing for making your breast-form pop out over the top of your bra, especially when you get up suddenly to talk to a neighbour! You need to make sure it's firmly in place before you start. They all said how careful they were of their hands to avoid infection, especially Jackie who had mild lymphoedema (see Chapter 8).

Breast reconstruction

Breast reconstruction is the replacement of the breast tissue removed by the surgeon with a silicone sac (bag) or with muscle from your back or abdomen. It is most often required after mastectomy, but sometimes it is used to deal with a defect left after lumpectomy. Breast reconstruction is a major, though not a dangerous, operation.

Expect a degree of discomfort as your body gets used to the implant in your chest – and it may take some time for normal sensation in your skin to return. It is difficult to make the breasts a perfect match, but in a swimsuit or underneath clothes, your new breast will look like your own. If you put on weight and the normal breast gets bigger you may need a fill-up of your silicone implant.

If you have breast reconstruction immediately while you are still under general anaesthetic from mastectomy, you wake up with your breast looking near to normal, but not all women want to have this done. Surgeons in the UK say that if they wait for the mastectomy to heal, only 5–10% of women will then ask for breast reconstruction. However, by that time it means another operation, more time off work and another stay in hospital. When breast reconstruction has been offered to all women having a mastectomy, up to 50% chose to have it. Whether you want immediate reconstruction or think you may want it later, you should discuss the options with the surgeon before you have your operation. You can always decide to have reconstruction months, or even years, later. If you have radiotherapy, you may need to wait for up to a year for the part of your chest which was treated to settle down, and before it is suitable for further surgery.

Breast reconstruction is available under the NHS provided your surgeon thinks you are suitable and there are no medical reasons why you shouldn't have it. If the surgeon seems to be unwilling to perform the operation for reasons other than medical ones, you can ask for a second opinion. Immediate reconstruction is usually carried out by a team including a breast surgeon and a plastic surgeon. It is therefore more complicated to arrange, and you may be discouraged from having it in a busy NHS department. You need to be persistent. If you decide to have your breast reconstruction carried out privately, you can expect to pay several thousand pounds.

If you decide you want breast reconstruction, talk to your breast-care nurse or contact BCC. Ask to meet a woman who has had the operation and is willing to show you what a reconstructed breast looks like.

Breast implants

A prosthesis is an artificial substitute for a part of the body. The term covers dentures (artificial teeth), as well as breast tissue substitutes, whether a breast-form inserted into your bra, or a silicone bag inserted under the skin and muscle of your chest. When prostheses are placed inside the body they are referred to as implants.

There are pros and cons for breast implants. A breast-form or external prosthesis may slip or get damaged or be obvious in some way to others. An implant appears more natural, but a fairly major operation is required. The implant sits quite high up on the chest wall, so you may need to have the other (normal) breast reduced in size or lifted to match.

Much research on implants has been carried out to find materials that are inert in the body and produce no irritation in the immediate area or harmful effects elsewhere in the body. Silicone sacs have been widely used, but reports of auto-immune diseases in women with silicone implants have made doctors more cautious.

However, a recent study carried out in the UK found no evidence of harmful effects – and the same material has been used successfully for many years for artificial joints and heart valves. If you are worried about side-effects from a silicone implant, your surgeon may recommend that a flap of your own tissue is used instead.

Implants beneath the skin

A plastic silicone 'envelope' is filled with silicone gel and placed under your skin through a horizontal cut through the lower part of your breast or in the crease below it. The implant feels soft and moves like a real breast. Sometimes a large amount of fibrous tissue (scar tissue) forms around the implant, making the breast feel hard and tight, and you may need a further operation to insert a new one. This operation is also carried out for normal women wanting bigger breasts and for women at high risk of breast cancer who choose to have mastectomy as a preventative measure. You may need a small implant in your normal breast if it looks a bit tired and droopy compared with your new breast.

Implants beneath the muscle

Some surgeons feel it is better to place the implant under the muscle of the chest wall. Should there be a recurrence of your cancer, it would be easier to detect than if there were a silicone sac over it. One disadvantage is that the implant can move when your muscle contracts. Radical mastectomy is rarely performed nowadays, but women who had this operation will have had their chest muscle removed. They can therefore only have implants under the skin.

Expanding silicone implants

Insertion of a simple implant as described above is only suitable for small to medium breasts – A to B cup fittings. Where the implant needs to be larger than that, the skin and underlying tissues may be too tight for the plastic surgeon to insert a suitable silicone prosthesis. The tissues are therefore stretched to make enough room by one of three methods.

1. An inflatable silicone implant with a one way valve is inserted under the chest muscle, with the patient under general anaesthetic. Each week, saline (sterile salt solution) is injected into the bag though the valve. When the breast is slightly larger than the normal one, the valve is removed. The breast is then left to settle down for three months or so and then a permanent silicone prosthesis is inserted under general anaesthetic.
2. A permanent but deflated silicone bag with a valve attached is inserted into the chest wall. The sac is expanded in the same way as in the first method, followed by a waiting period of about three months. The valve is then removed under local anaesthetic.
3. The implant is replaced as the tissue expands. This gives better control over the final shape, but requires more operations.

Side-effects of breast reconstruction with a silicone implant

Breast reconstruction is a major operation, and you may feel as tired and let down as after any operation. A few women have trouble with infection, and some have quite a lot of pain and discomfort. In some, the implant gets encased in hard scar tissue and may need to be replaced. In the UK, studies have failed to show that silicone causes auto-immune diseases, such as rheumatoid arthritis.

Reconstruction using your own muscle and skin

A great deal of experience in reconstructing parts of the body was gained in World War II, in repairing wounds received in battle. Techniques for moving skin and underlying tissue from other parts of the body were perfected and adapted for use in peacetime life.

Skin, underlying fat and connective tissue can be swung round to your mastectomy site either from your back or your abdomen. Most often it remains attached to the donor site on the back or abdomen by a tube of tissue (called the pedicle). When the graft has 'taken' and developed its own blood supply, the pedicle is cut free and the wound sewn up. A newer, more complex method allows the piece of skin and muscle to be removed completely from the donor site. The graft is placed on the chest wall and the surgeon connects the blood vessels by microsurgery, rather than waiting for new blood vessels to grow to nourish the tissue.

The flap taken from the back is called a Latissimus Dorsi flap, after the name of the main muscle contained in it. Its disadvantage is that it may not have enough bulk to construct a large breast, and a silicone implant may still be needed as well. The abdominal flap (the Transverse Rectus Abdominus Musculo-cutaneous flap – TRAM flap) has the advantage of taking tissue away from the abdomen where so many of us would like some removed. Both methods leave a scar at the donor site; they are both major operations requiring at least a week in hospital and are prone to minor complications.

False nipples and nipple reconstruction

Women who have had a conventional mastectomy have an area of overlying skin and the nipple removed. After your breast is reconstructed, it won't therefore have a nipple. In addition, lumpectomy with removal of the nipple is now offered to women who have cancer under the nipple, instead of mastectomy. Many women in this situation are not fussed about being without a nipple, and a bra with a horizontal seam disguises the fact that one breast has a nipple and the other hasn't.

If you aren't happy, you can get an off-the-shelf stick-on nipple or even have one custom-made to match the other (BCC will send details – see Useful addresses).

Alternatively, you can have a further operation in which a permanent nipple is constructed from a part of the normal side, if it is large enough, or from skin taken from elsewhere. This is usually carried out at least six months after the main breast reconstruction has settled down. The operation requires a good deal of skill and results may not be perfect.

11

Complementary medicine

Complementary and conventional treatment

Until quite recently the view of orthodox doctors was that complementary medicine was all very well as long as it didn't do you any harm, but that it was for cranks. It was called 'alternative medicine', and was offered instead of, not as well as, conventional treatment. Those seeking alternative therapies would give up conventional treatment. As a result, some breast cancers grew unchecked to a stage where treatment was very difficult, and this coloured the view of cancer specialists.

Doctors are now more open-minded about complementary medicine. Many feel that certain complementary therapies are of benefit to the patient, and some conventionally trained doctors practice one or more of them. The emphasis is on using these therapies side by side with conventional medicine, hence the newer name of complementary medicine. If your doctor advises against a particular type, you should think seriously about using it. If you think your doctor is just being old-fashioned, ask for a second opinion – but it is unwise to abandon your regular treatment without very careful consideration. There are some extreme diets, for example, which would not be recommended by orthodox doctors, nor perhaps by other more moderate complementary practitioners; nor would other way-out treatments like injection of cells from unborn animals. The treatments reviewed here are compatible with radiotherapy and chemotherapy, and some are offered in NHS cancer units.

Many women with breast cancer try complementary therapies. The extra personal care so often provided by complementary therapists can make all the difference to how you feel, to the quality of your life. However there is as yet no scientific proof that any of them can cure cancer.

If you want to give up conventional treatment, it is your choice, but you should not stop your treatment without discussing the risks involved with your doctor. You need to find a doctor who will not just wash his hands of you but make you feel you can return for orthodox treatment if you so wish.

The initial treatment of primary breast cancer

A hospital trained doctor would insist that the first line of treatment for primary breast cancer must be conventional. They may have seen the horrific results of persisting with herbal or other remedies while the cancer continued to grow.

Practitioners of complementary medicine complain that women don't come to see them until they have widespread cancer and conventional medicine has nothing more to offer. They would like cancer patients to come to them much earlier. Certainly some of the therapies are helpful to women whose breast cancer is completely removed and who have no evidence of spread.

I asked some homoeopathic practitioners whether they would treat primary breast cancer without the patient also having hospital treatment. They replied that it was the patient's choice, and told me stories of GPs trying to frighten their patients into having surgery by recounting all the possible unpleasant outcomes. I would find it unethical not to try to persuade a woman to have her breast cancer removed or treated by radiotherapy or chemotherapy – though perhaps not by terrifying her – and some complementary therapists would feel the same.

Holistic medicine and taking control

Holistic medicine is treatment of the patient as a whole, not just the treatment of their disease. Conventionally-trained doctors are aware of the need to treat the whole person, but those who practise complementary medicine spend a great deal more time talking to patients about their life style and problems. The constraints of time under the NHS make it more difficult to do this.

Many women feel they are treated like 'things' when they have cancer, and some would like to feel more in control. However, they and their relatives can feel let down or guilty if the cancer recurs or spreads while they have been trying to follow a complementary regime or special diet. They may have been using visualization, telling their cancer cells to die, and may have been made to feel that their cancer is in some way their own fault. If only they hadn't lived their lives in the way they had, not eaten meat, or not reacted to stress in a defensive way, their cancer might not have occurred. But 75% of breast cancer patients have no proven risk factors. At present, the best way we have of reducing death from breast cancer is to remove tumours when they are still small. We would all like to prevent breast cancer, but as yet we don't know how to do so.

There is no doubt that some complementary therapies improve the quality of our lives. One study of women with widespread secondary breast cancer showed that those given counselling, invited to attend weekly meetings and encouraged to live life fully, survived longer than those not offered this, though they were not cured.

Other studies have confirmed the benefit of this 'psychosocial' help to the wellbeing of patients, – how they feel about their disease and how they cope with pain and the side effects of treatment – but none, so far, have confirmed the increase in length of survival, though further research is under way.

There is a feeling (see the section on stories and statistics in Chapter 3) that cancer patients who have a fighting spirit do better, but studies proving this remain to be published. I suspect that some cancers produce a substance which makes us depressed and feel we will never get better. It is possible that those cancers which are going to respond to treatment do not produce these substances, so it may be easier to be optimistic and have a fighting spirit if your cancer is one of these.

However, some very depressed cancer patients are cured and some very optimistic ones are not.

Evaluating complementary therapies

There are claims of complementary practitioners achieving 'miracle' cures in patients given no hope by conventional doctors. They say that these are not published in the medical press so doctors never hear about them. However, most cancer patients have also been treated with radiotherapy or chemotherapy, and it would be difficult to be sure that their cure wasn't a late result of that treatment. Some cancers get smaller or stop growing without treatment. There are plenty of examples of patients who have survived cancer with neither conventional nor complementary treatment, when their doctors said they had only months to live. Dr Bloom studied the records of 250 patients with breast cancer seen at the Middlesex Hospital in London from 1805 to 1933. All had cancer which was advanced or had spread elsewhere in the body, and none were treated, either because they refused treatment or for other reasons. Nearly one in five (18.4%) survived five years and nearly one in 25 (3.6%) was still alive ten years later. It is in this context that complementary therapies (and conventional treatment) must be assessed. Doctors and patients alike are wary of charlatans, 'quack doctors', and you should keep clear of anyone who promises very high cure rates. If any treatment were so remarkably successful, orthodox doctors would adopt it at once.

For a new treatment to be adopted by the conventional medical profession, it has to be tested very stringently and compared with treatments already available. This means that when a pharmaceutical company brings out a new drug it is tested against the old one to make sure it really is better, not just newer and more expensive. Doctors are well aware of what is called the 'placebo effect' (see Chapter 3). We all feel good when someone takes an interest in us. That we are being treated at all can make us feel better, even if the pills we are given contain just chalk or some other harmless but inactive substance.

The effects of some types of complementary medicine, like those based on meditation, are very difficult to measure, though not impossible. If they are to be adopted widely and given a place in regular cancer treatment, complementary therapies must be tested in the same stringent way as conventional treatment. Some of those recommending complementary therapies suggest that doctors do not accept their methods because they are motivated only by greed or envy. This is not true.

Once a positive report, based on a sound clinical trial, is published, new treatments for cancer are adopted surprisingly quickly, even in a country as conservative as ours.

I feel very strongly that if complementary therapies prolong life or actually cure cancer, it is the duty of complementary practitioners to carry out scientifically acceptable trials and prove that their methods work. Research is never easy. If controlled trials comparing one treatment with another were carried out these therapies could be funded by the NHS and could be made available to all of us in general hospitals, not in just a few specialised centres.

Types of complementary medicine

Most types of complementary medicine are very ancient, and some forms of conventional treatment, like the use of drugs originally derived from plants, are firmly rooted in them. In some countries, particularly in the East, they form the mainstay of the treatment of a wide variety of diseases.

Some complementary therapies are available in cancer units or at your GP practice. They are safely carried out during conventional therapy, provided the person carrying them out is properly trained and you have discussed it with your specialist or your GP. You will be discouraged from strict diets which could lead to nutritional deficiency, and from vigorous massage of your operation site. The time should have passed when the response of doctors to patients wanting to try out other methods of treatment was to refuse to carry on looking after them.

Acupuncture

Acupuncture is an ancient Chinese technique. In cancer treatment it is mainly used for the relief of pain and tension, and the prevention of nausea. The theory behind it is that the life-force or *Chi* flows along pathways called meridians. Diseases are thought to appear if these meridians become blocked, and acupuncture is thought to divert this energy and treat the blockages.

Sterile needles are used for each patient, so that there is no possibility of passing on AIDS or other infections. Unless you have experienced the technique you may imagine a needle a foot long and as thick as a knitting needle. In fact, the needles most commonly used are less than one inch in length and so fine that you can only just feel the prick.

Scientific experiments on the use of acupuncture have shown that it releases endorphins, the body's own substances which behave very like morphine. You may be quite severely hurt in a game or in a battle and not feel a thing until afterwards; the endorphins released by wounding have anaesthetised you against the pain. In some countries, such as China, acupuncture is used to produce enough anaesthesia for surgery.

The response to acupuncture is very individual. It rarely works on people who are very apprehensive or don't really want it, but have been persuaded to try it by relatives or friends. Up to 10% of people, especially children, are very strong responders; 10–30% do not respond at all or find acupuncture makes them feel worse. If you do get any benefit it is likely to continue or even improve over further treatments.

Aromatherapy

Aromatherapy is treatment using various aromatic oils which are extracted from plants. They contain active substances some of which can be absorbed through the skin. Application by massage is the best-known method, but the oils can also be sniffed, added to bath water or even taken by mouth. Aromatherapy is used as one type of beauty therapy, and like other types of massage is relaxing and soothing.

Because of the oils used, it is thought by its practitioners to have specific healing properties. You need to ask whether the oils used are suitable for cancer patients.

Art and music therapy

Taking part in art and music classes makes you feel good, even if you are just a beginner. I find it helps to take me out of myself and forget my cancer.

If you are like me, you were told at school that you were so useless at art that you could be excused. It was not until I read Betty Edward's book (see Further reading) which claims that we can all draw that I tried going to Art Classes. Though I am no Picasso, it gives me great pleasure, and I find I can draw and paint.

Art therapists encourage their patients to draw themselves, their cancer and their treatment. They talk the drawings through with their patients and help them to come to terms with their cancer. They say they can see a difference in the drawings produced as the patient comes to understand their disease and their reactions to it.

Some proponents of art and music therapy claim participation will help you defeat cancer.

Autogenic training

Autogenic training, a technique for dealing with stress by simple mental exercises, was evolved in the 1930s by Dr Schultz and further developed by Dr Luthe. Its aim is to induce mental and physical relaxation, and improve communication between the two sides of the brain, and the nervous systems. It is said to be of value in helping women deal with the problems of breast cancer.

Diet

Many women feel better if they change to a healthier diet, with more fruit and fibre and less meat and animal fat. The view of modern medicine is that a healthier life-style is desirable and may well prevent a number of cancers. For example, it is unusual for non-smokers to develop lung cancer, or non-alcoholics in developed countries to get liver cancer. Similarly cancer of the bowel is rare in countries where people live on a high fibre diet. If we look at all women with breast cancer, a larger number than would be expected are overweight. If a more natural diet includes maintenance of a normal weight, it might help to prevent breast cancer, though there is not yet any evidence to support this.

Conventional doctors would not support the use of any diet that severely restricts your calorie intake. One of the effects of cancer is to make you lose weight, at least when it spreads elsewhere in the body. Diets like those which are strictly vegetarian and attempt to use only organically-grown foods are often expensive and difficult to keep up. Not everyone is convinced of the value of organically-grown food. There are high rates of some cancers, like liver cancer and cancers of childhood, in countries where farming is very primitive and all food is organically grown.

Herbal medicines

Diseases have been treated with plant extracts since ancient times, and numerous herbals (books of herbal remedies) became widely available shortly after printing was invented. One aspect of herbal medicine is a belief in the importance of the patient's 'vital force', and herbalists will take a full medical history, and try to restore the body's balance to normal.

A number of conventional drugs – like digitalis from the foxglove for heart disease, and vincristine, the anti-cancer drug, from *Vinca rosea*, a member of the periwinkle family – were originally extracted from plants. Since plant extracts contain highly active ingredients, herbal medicines must be taken with great care, under the supervision of a trained herbalist and with the knowledge of your conventional doctor.

Homoeopathic medicine

Drugs have been used homoeopathically for many thousands of years, but the discipline of homoeopathy was established in the eighteenth century by a German physician, Dr Hahnemann. He described the principle on which homoeopathy is based: that drugs which cause symptoms may be used in tiny quantities to treat those same symptoms. For example an extract of onion (which makes your eyes sore and runny) may be used to treat a runny nose or sore eyes. Unlike conventional medicine, homoeopathic drugs are tested on healthy people to see whether they produce similar symptoms to the one to be treated. These are called 'provings', but they are not controlled trials and substances are not initially tested on cancer patients.

Most homoeopathic remedies are derived from plant sources, quite a few from mineral sources, and a small number are of animal origin. Unlike conventional medicines, they are dispensed in very low concentrations so that there may only be a few molecules of the drug in each dose. During their dilution they are shaken repeatedly. This 'succussion' is considered an important and integral part of the preparation.

It is difficult to conceive of drugs being active in the minute quantities used in homoeopathic medicine, often in sub-molecular amounts. This means that each dose of the medicine you take may contain less than one molecule of the active substance, in other words, none at all. However, there have been controlled trials showing that some such remedies work, at least in the treatment of certain diseases, like asthma.

In the past, homoeopathic practitioners were content to rely on provings, toxicological studies (studies of the poisonous effect of drugs) and clinical experience. They felt that it was wrong to deprive any of their patients of treatment in order to carry out clinical trials. In several centres, however, studies which would meet conventional criteria are beginning to be carried out.

Although some conventionally trained doctors use homoeopathic remedies, many would have reservations about homoeopathic medicines, and you should certainly take no drugs without informing your doctor. If your homoeopath is properly trained, he or she will want to contact your GP before prescribing any medicines.

A variety of homoeopathic medicines are available to help with the nausea associated with chemotherapy, and with anxiety and pain.

Iscador

The anthroposophical philosophical movement was founded by Rudolf Steiner, who, in 1920, suggested that Iscador, an extract of mistletoe, be used in the treatment of cancer. Its use is based on the fact that mistletoe is a parasite on other plants.

Anthroposophical practitioners believe that, like the mistletoe, cancer is a parasite on humans – though of course cancers are quite different from a parasite. They are composed of our own cells though these are abnormal. (The one exception is the tumour in women derived from the placenta, a choriocarcinoma. These cells are derived from the foetus not the mother.) Claims for the success of Iscador are difficult to evaluate and to the observer seem to be too high to be likely.

Massage

Body massage has an old and hallowed place in the treatment of aches and pains. We almost automatically rub a sore place, and one of the of the first things we hear is 'Mummy will rub it better'. Anyone who has had massage whether as part of beauty treatment, for rheumatic aches and pains or for whatever reason, can testify to its benefit. Having your shoulders and neck massaged after a hard day is one of life's pleasures. Even if you don't have any sore places, massage can make you feel relaxed and more at peace with yourself.

> Tina said that for her, massage was a life saver. After surgery and the removal of her axillary lymph nodes, her arm felt heavy and not part of her body. Massage helped to re-integrate it into her body.

Any area which has had radiotherapy should not be massaged, and it is wise to avoid the operation site. There is no evidence to suggest that massage can make cancer spread, though the emphasis is on gentle therapy. Vigorous massage of any kind may not be advisable for some cancer patients.

Some people don't like being touched by strangers and for them massage may not be suitable, though if they want to try it, a partner or friend can be taught some basic techniques.

Meditation

Meditation got a bad press at the time of the hippies when Transcendental Meditation was all the thing. Meditation now has a wide following in the West, as well as in the East where many of the techniques evolved. The aim of meditation is to improve the quality of your life by switching off stress pathways and guiding your thoughts towards health. It is difficult at first to stop thinking about your problems, but you can gradually learn to do so. Techniques include imagining pleasant places – a quiet cove by the sea, a hilltop in spring sunshine – to help you to relax and think quietly. Some women find meditation of value in coming to terms with their cancer. Many adult education centres run meditation sessions, or you may be able to borrow suitable tapes from your local library.

Reflexology

Reflexology is a specific form of massage, usually of the feet but sometimes of the hands. Reflexology is based on the belief that the body is reflected (represented) in different parts of the foot or hand, with, for example, the head represented in the thumb or big toe. Its practitioners believe that, by applying pressure to one area of the foot or hand, they can induce well-being and relaxation in the part it reflects.

This is said to influence the relationship between different organs of the body.

Cancer patients who do not feel up to body massage often find massage of the feet or hands relaxing and helpful.

Relaxation

If you have ever been to a relaxation class, whether in an antenatal department or for after-work relaxation, you will know how good it makes you feel. There may be relaxation classes at the hospital where you were treated, or your GP may run a relaxation class.

The aim of relaxation is to quieten down all mental activity and achieve relief from tension and anxiety, usually while listening to soft speech by the therapist or on a tape-recording.

Shiatsu (Japanese massage)

Shiatsu literally means finger pressure. It is the Japanese method of accessing acupuncture points and meridians, and it is sometimes referred to as acupressure, or acupuncture without needles. Its practitioners may also use pressure from hands, elbows, knees and feet. Shiatsu is performed on clothed patients and some people prefer it for this reason. It is available in some cancer centres and, like acupuncture, is used in the treatment of pain and tension.

Spiritual healing

Many religions have a place for healing by laying on of hands, and some people believe they can cure by touching cancer patients, even from a distance. Those treated by healers often say they have a feeling of warmth at the site where they are touched. If you like the idea of trying spiritual healing you do not have to subscribe to any particular religion – though you may prefer to ask to see someone of your own faith.

Anne was a hard-headed businesswoman whose cancer was picked up on a mammogram when it was quite large. She had radiotherapy and then chemotherapy to shrink it, and was pleasurably surprised to find that her oncologist didn't try to belittle her when she rather shamefacedly said she had been to see a healer. She said she had a feeling of warmth and comfort which made her feel good.

Visualization

Carl and Stephanie Simonton introduced the idea of visualization in the 1970s. They teach that by creating images of your cancer cells in your mind's eye or in your drawings you can destroy them. They used images of the body's white cells as dogs attacking the cancer cells which are seen as broken-up hamburgers, or of fish eating greyish cancer cells. Some people imagine their white blood cells as knights on horseback riding off to kill the 'baddies', the cancer cells. Others are happier thinking of their white cells as dustmen taking the malignant cells out to the rubbish bin.

Visualization has been recommended both for preventing your cancer from recurring or spreading, or for destroying it once it has spread. There are anecdotal stories (see Chapter 3) of cancer patients recovering from widespread cancer using these techniques, but as yet there is no hard evidence, and no controlled trials have been reported. If it makes you feel better, try it. People who can naturally see pictures in their mind's eye find the technique easier than those who think more in words. The danger is that patients may feel guilty and responsible if their cancer recurs. They may feel they have just not been trying hard enough. This is self-destructive and harmful, and should be strongly discouraged.

Vitamin supplements

Supplements of vitamin C, beta carotene, which is converted to vitamin A in the body, vitamin B, selenium, and zinc are included in some complementary cancer diets. Their benefit is unproven, and you probably get enough of these in a normal, mixed diet. It can be harmful to take excessive amounts of certain vitamins, like vitamins A and D. Vitamin E, which is related chemically to oestrogen, may not be a good idea for breast cancer patients. However controlled trials are being carried out on the effect of taking extra selenium and retinoids, which are converted into vitamin A in the body. If you are having chemotherapy, you should not take vitamin supplements without consulting your doctor in case they interact with your cytotoxic drugs.

Writing

If you keep a diary you can see how your mood improves day by day. If you feel miserable, you can look back and see what you did to help yourself get over the 'blues' before. A diary kept for your eyes only lets you admit that having cancer gets you down. You can write that you feel hard-done-by, and that you'd rather it were someone else who had it not you. It can make you feel much better to express nasty thoughts which you feel you ought not to have, and wouldn't dream of mentioning to anyone.

Some cancer patients find that they get pleasure and release from writing poetry, even though they haven't written any since their school-days.

Yoga

Yoga is a well-known combination of relaxation, breathing techniques and exercise. It is taught that *pranayama* (control of the breath) promotes circulation and improves oxygenation of the cells of the body, increases strength and augments *prana*, the life-force. The positions taken up in yoga are said to train the nervous and immune systems to work together to improve function. *Mantras* are healing sounds which are chanted to aid the process.

Does complementary medicine work?

There are not yet sufficient studies to determine whether any form of complementary medicine is effective in prolonging survival or in preventing cancer recurrence. If it makes you feel better and more positive towards your cancer and your life as a whole, it seems reasonable to suppose it will increase your chances of doing well. There is an interest in carrying out scientific trials of some of the types of therapy mentioned to seek independent proof of their efficacy. We await the results with interest.

The cost of complementary medicine

Some types of complementary medicine are available in hospital or at your GP's practice free of charge. Some are available at local cancer self-help groups (Cancerlink maintains a list – see Useful addresses). Local groups usually expect some contribution, and treatment from a private practitioner can work out expensive, as can some diets. Any treatment on a one-to-one basis is likely to be more expensive than treatment in groups.

Arrange a consultation and see how you get on with the practitioner. Ask how much it is all going to cost and don't be afraid to say 'No'. If you can, take a friend and see how they react. Are they convinced? If it looks as if it will make you feel good, go for it (for list of practitioners, see address of Institute of Complementary Medicine in Useful addresses).

12

The psychological aspects
of breast cancer

When women (and men) find they have breast cancer, they often feel terribly alone and vulnerable. We are used to discussing our physical problems, but it's much more difficult to admit to our fears and doubts. We feel we should be strong and able to deal with the psychological aspects of cancer ourselves, especially if we have been running a home and looking after a family.

First suspicions

Perhaps the worst time is when you suspect you may have breast cancer but don't know for sure. You have found a lump, or you notice that your nipple looks odd on one side, or you have had a routine mammogram and are asked to attend an assessment clinic. Everyone around you seems to be cheerful and happy, while you have this thing hanging over you. Every day that you have to wait for an appointment or for the results seems like an age.

Many women think that breast cancer is a death sentence. They delay going to the doctor because they feel that it is hopeless and that they will not be helped by the sort of mutilating operation their grandmothers had. They don't realise that breast cancer is eminently treatable, and their very delay makes mastectomy rather than lumpectomy more likely. Breast reconstruction is possible after mastectomy or lumpectomy (see Chapter 10) and for those who don't want breast reconstruction, breast-forms are now very good.

I am always surprised at how little my non-medical friends know about breast cancer. There needs to be more publicity about the good news. The number of deaths from breast cancer in this country is finally falling. The five-year survival rate of women with small cancers, which have not yet spread to the lymph glands, is 84%. Taking all stages of breast cancer survival is 62%, while even in women with widespread cancer, five-year survival is nearly 20%.

Not every woman feels devastated. Some always expected that they would get breast cancer one day, and it is almost a relief when it finally develops.

Judith came from a breast cancer family. Her mother had died of breast cancer and so had an aunt. There were even rumours that her grandmother had also died of breast cancer in Eastern Europe. When Judith was 62 she found a lump in her breast. She was philosophical. 'I knew I'd get it one day,' she said. 'I am lucky I have lived to see my children grow up.' Foolishly, having breast cancer hanging over her head, she had avoided regular mammography, thinking that she was fated anyhow. Instead of reporting her lump as soon as she found it, she went on holiday first and travelled the world. She wasn't surprised to be told her cancer had spread to her lymph glands but she took mastectomy and chemotherapy in her stride. She doesn't expect to live to be 82 (the present average expectation of life for women in the UK who reach 60), but she is grateful for the life she has had so far. Her family finds it difficult to forgive her for not catching her cancer when it was small enough to treat with a hope of cure.

Women who have tiny cancers found on mammography may feel shattered at the news but some, like Sonia, feel their regular attendance for screening was rewarded by finding a cancer while it was still small.

Sonia worked for a large company which arranged for their female staff to be seen regularly at a Well Woman Clinic. She had had regular mammography since before her fiftieth birthday, and had accepted that one day a cancer might be found. When a small cancer showed up on her second mammogram, she was pleased that her check-ups had paid off. Her cancer was removed by lumpectomy and found to be less than one centimetre in diameter with no nodes involved. She hopes to live to a ripe old age.

We suddenly find we know almost nothing about the disease we suspect we may have. None of our friends knows anything about breast cancer either, and our GP seems evasive. Sometimes that is because he himself cannot be sure whether we have cancer or not – it is difficult to be certain until either an FNA or biopsy is carried out (see Chapter 6).

The diagnosis confirmed

Some women feel almost relieved when they are told they have cancer, and all the waiting and worrying are over. Many then want to have their treatment over and done with as soon as possible.

The cytologist told me I definitely had breast cancer after he had looked at my FNA. When I then talked to the surgeon, he already knew the result, and said I could come in at the end of the week. I said I would as soon have it out on the kitchen table as wait one more day. I really wanted my cancer out of me. Fortunately he was able to find a bed for the next day. I went into work first and carried on as normal. When it came to the last case before lunch, the diagnosis wasn't clear and we had to order some extra tests. I quite enjoyed shocking the young male, junior doctor, telling him he would have to take the new slides to one of my colleagues as I was going in that afternoon to have my own breast cancer removed!

Different reactions to the knowledge of having breast cancer and – how it might affect you – are described later in this chapter (pages 126–8).

The prospect of mastectomy

In a society like ours, with Page Three pin-ups and advertisements using women in sexy underwear to sell anything and everything, it is not surprising that some of us feel that, in losing a breast, we have lost our femininity, our very essence.

Margaret felt so bad at the thought of losing her breast that she decided that if the choice were mastectomy or nothing, she would opt for nothing and be prepared to die of her cancer. She said her new, younger husband was brilliant. 'I realized he wanted me, myself, as opposed to wanting ''it'', my breast.'

Others have a different view.

Eizabeth, an unmarried woman in her late 60s, had a matter-of-fact attitude towards her mastectomy. 'I suppose it would have been worse,' she said, 'if I'd been married. And I was always small anyhow.' She had had a rheumaticky shoulder for some time, and the most comfortable position in bed was to lie on the other side. Never having heard that an inverted nipple may be a sign of cancer, she ignored the fact that the nipple on that side had become drawn in. She assumed it was due to lying on it. When she finally went to see her GP about her arthritis, he examined her thoroughly. He noticed her inverted nipple and found a small underlying lump. She was seen quickly at her local hospital and told she had to have a mastectomy rather than lumpectomy because the tumour was under the nipple. Like most postmenopausal women, she was prescribed Tamoxifen, to help

119

prevent recurrence and spread. Elizabeth thinks she should have been warned that the drug might make her feel sick and dizzy and get swollen feet. A year later these side-effects have gone and she feels fine.

Although some elderly patients, and those women who are not sexually active, may feel this way, there are plenty of older women who feel badly about losing a breast. They are just as much in need of sympathetic counselling as younger women.

If you are recommended mastectomy, remember that you are a person, and you are not just your breast. It is horrible to think of having a leg or arm amputated, but no-one would suggest that you were not a woman if such surgery were required. Why is a breast different? Even if you have to have your whole breast removed you can have a breast-form to put in your bra, and people will not be able to tell you've had surgery. It is up to us to educate our loved ones that we are still women whether we have one breast or two, or none, and learn to feel that way ourselves.

The prospect of lumpectomy

Agreeing to lumpectomy is not all plain sailing either. We may worry that some cancer may be left behind, that the subsequent radiotherapy will make us feel ill or that our hair will fall out (it doesn't), or dread having chemotherapy. We may worry what our breast will look like with a big lump taken out of it, or we may not be too bothered.

I am not sure why, perhaps because I had resigned myself to mastectomy when I found my cancer, but the appearance of my breast was not one of my major concerns. I thought the survival of women with breast cancer was much worse than it is. My excuse was that I worked in a cancer hospital for four years, and as a pathologist, I saw only women who had died of their disease. I just hadn't looked up the data carefully until I started to carry out research for this book. My cancer was small enough to be removed locally, and I think the scar that has healed to a fine white line is rather decorative. I tease the surgeon who did the operation by saying that my left breast is nicer with a tuck in it and can't I have the other one adjusted to match. If I were younger and went topless on public beaches, I think I might try to persuade him.

Patients who are about to have a lumpectomy rather than mastectomy may miss out on pre-operative counselling, especially if their hospital does not have a breast-care nurse. Though they don't have the worry of a mastectomy they are still scared about having surgery, especially if this is their first hospital admission. They have the same fear of dying from their disease as do the women who are to have mastectomy.

Often the same amount of time is not spent with them, reassuring them and dealing with their fears, because they are not going to have a mastectomy.

Facing up to having cancer

To judge from articles in the popular press you would think the most important thing for women with breast cancer is the thought of mastectomy. For many, the thought that they might die of their disease is far worse. Some women are able to respond by regarding every day as a bonus. They can take a look at their family relationships and their work and re-appraise both. They start hobbies they've always wanted to try, visit faraway places and determine to live their life to the full.

Fortunate couples may find a closeness they have never before experienced.

Looking at your breast the first time

Breast wounds often look red and rather horrid to begin with, and then settle down to a thin white line which is hardly noticeable. Some women would rather have the breast-care nurse (if there is one) or a staff nurse with them when they look at their breast for the first time. Whatever it looks like, its appearance will improve as the scar shrinks and gets paler. If it looks ugly to you when it has thoroughly healed, you can ask your surgeon to tidy up the scar.

Letting your partner see your scar

While you are still in hospital you can ask the breast-care nurse or staff nurse to be with you when you show your partner your breast for the first time. Whatever your breast looks like, the chances are they've seen much worse on television or at the cinema!

> Joyce had a loving, caring husband. He was as supportive as anyone could wish while she was waiting for an appointment to see the surgeon and then waiting to have her lumpectomy. Finally she got home and had her first bath. She asked Len to come in. Before he could stop himself he had blurted out, 'Looks just like Frankenstein,' never having seen a surgical wound with stitch marks close up. Joyce burst into tears and wished she was back in the ward. Len felt terrible. He didn't know what to say at first, but then he said what was needed to reassure her.

Many women feel great in the busy atmosphere of the ward, being jollied along by the nurses and other patients. When they come home it is like when you take your baby home for the first time: you are on your own.

My youngest child was born prematurely in 1967 and had a severe breathing problem from which she nearly died. I can still recall the feeling of panic and isolation when I finally left the security and companionship of the hospital ward, carrying my tiny daughter, still too small to be bathed in anything larger than a hand-basin.

Sex after breast surgery

There is no medical reason why you shouldn't have sex after mastectomy or lumpectomy. However, many women do have problems after their operation, and this is not confined to women who have had mastectomy. Even after lumpectomy, your breast may be tender to touch for some time and the nipple may be unpleasantly sensitive for weeks or months. If you are having chemotherapy, some days you may feel awful and it's hard to think about sex. If your relationship is a bit rocky anyhow, this may be the last straw and it may break up. On the other hand, some couples find that a disaster like breast cancer brings them closer together.

Men who feel a bit low are often cheered up by having sex and seem to be able to do so at a mainly physical level. It is also a way in which they express their love and care. It is often different for women, who may be worried about having cancer or about whether their partner is going to hurt their tender breast or be disgusted by it, and it may be impossible for them to relax enough to enjoy, or even to want sex. You can feel so sure your partner will reject you after mastectomy that you turn away before you can be hurt by that rejection. Some partners are afraid of touching the operation side in case they do some damage, and they need reassuring that, when it is no longer tender, they can do no harm. They may feel that they should not be forcing their attentions on a woman who has 'been through all that'. Both partners need to be patient. As women come to terms with their feelings, it gets easier.

Tamoxifen and sex

Vaginal dryness is a very common side-effect of the anti-oestrogen drug Tamoxifen, (see Chapter 9) so that intercourse is uncomfortable or even painful without the use of a lubricating jelly. Ask the chemist about some of the newer ones. They really seem to work. In some women Tamoxifen also reduces the desire for sex, making matters even worse – as well as causing embarrassing hot flushes and sudden sweats. Large studies have shown that Tamoxifen reduces the death rate from breast cancer, recurrence and cancer in the other breast, so you will be encouraged to go on taking your tablets. Most of the side-effects get better with time. You and your partner must be patient and ask advice from your oncologist, the breast-care nurse or one of the cancer help organisations (see Useful addresses).

Partners, family and friends

Learning the diagnosis and undergoing treatment is a stressful experience, and relationships with partners, whether male or female, family and friends can become strained. There often seems to be a conspiracy in families – women not wanting their families to be told about their cancer, and relatives trying to keep the truth from the patient. Everyone should choose for themselves whether they want to know the facts or not, and it is up to health professionals to be aware of our right to know the truth if we want to. They should not be too responsive to our relatives' wishes to save us pain.

As young doctors in the late 1950s, we were discouraged from telling patients the truth. We used to refer to cancer by all sorts of medical names which the patients wouldn't understand. Nowadays unless a patient makes it clear they would rather not know, doctors believe in telling patients the truth. We all have things we need to put in order, if there's a chance we might die of our cancer, and it is unfair to deprive us of the chance to do so.

Women often feel bad about not being able to do all the housework, cooking and child-care that they did before. It may be especially difficult for those brought up at a time when men thought housework unfit for them. The person who takes over may be only too pleased to help out and show their love by doing something practical rather than just talking.

We'd like to think of ourselves as being supportive and caring, and we expect our families and friends to be the same. But they are not angels, and have the same feelings of 'Why me? Why my family or friend?' It is hard for them to realise how easily our feelings are hurt. We all want constant reassurance, but sometimes when they say 'Everything will be OK' and 'Don't worry,' we feel that they don't understand how serious cancer is. It is difficult for them to strike the right balance, especially if secretly they are terrified.

Some husbands and partners go completely to pieces. They feel guilty at being fit and well when their partner has cancer, or they may feel bitter about having to take on extra responsibilities. Some women find that they are having to support their husbands and families, to stop them worrying, rather than the other way round. It is often assumed that adolescent daughters will automatically take over running the house, even when there is a husband or partner, or older sons. It is not surprising that some daughters resent this imposition, and they are quite right to do so.

Women partners suffer the same anguish as male partners, and experience a similar range of feelings, perhaps sometimes worse because they can more readily imagine the loss of all or part of a breast. When the one with cancer is in hospital it may be difficult for her partner to show affection openly, and they may not be offered the same range of support and counselling services as a heterosexual couple.

It is often difficult to know what to do about telling children who are old enough to understand. Above all, they resent being kept in the dark. Painful as it is to be told the truth, your children would rather know.

Joanna said that the worst thing about her mother having cancer was that her family lied to her. She was told her mother had gone into hospital for something quite minor. The daughter of a family friend was in the same class and she found out from her. She felt terrible because she thought her mother was going to die, and felt let down by everyone. Why should strangers know things about her mother that she didn't?

I was just as bad.

One of my daughters teaches English in the north of Spain. I didn't want her to worry about me and preferred her not to know until after my operation. My elder son insisted on phoning her. She said how much she would have hated not to have been told. Of course she was worried and anxious, but she didn't feel left out just because she wasn't in England at the time.

Cancer families are rare, and most breast cancers are not familial, but mothers may feel guilty at having a disease they might have passed on to their daughters. Daughters may feel resentful at the thought their mother has compromised their future.

Sometimes people are so worried about saying the wrong thing to cancer patients that they avoid talking to them altogether. This can seem very hurtful – for example, when you return to work – but it all gets better with time.

Partners and families can ask for support and advice from cancer help lines. BCC has a partners' network; CancerLink can put gay women in touch with The Lesbian Network for women affected by cancer (see Useful addresses).

Thinking about cancer

I think about my cancer a lot, especially when I get twinges around the shoulder on that side or in my breast – and many other women do too.

> Brigit was a cheerful 38-year old woman with young children. Like many of us, she had been completely floored by the news that she had breast cancer. She had been to see her GP because she could feel a lump, and had been told there was nothing there. When she finally took herself to hospital and insisted on seeing someone, a tiny cancer was found. She was admitted within days for lumpectomy and axillary clearance.
>
> 'I don't think a day passes without me thinking about my cancer. Through the church I met a woman of my age who also had breast cancer. After having to keep a stiff upper lip in front of my husband, it was such a relief finding someone with similar experiences with whom I could talk about anything and admit how worried I get.'

Counselling

Cancer brings with it all sorts of unpleasant emotions like fear, anger, sadness and guilt. Talking through your problems with a counsellor, who will listen without interrupting and without telling you what to do, can be of tremendous help. Some counselling is carried out by the breast-care nurse while you are in hospital, but professional counselling may be most helpful for you and your family when you are discharged. Many women have strong feelings of guilt about their breast cancer.

You may have emotional and sexual problems which are difficult to discuss with your hospital doctor or GP. You may be able to have counselling on a one-to-one basis arranged by the hospital; some GPs have a trained counsellor attached to the practice.

Self-help groups

Almost all of us with breast cancer gain immensely from talking to other women with breast cancer. BCC (see Useful addresses) keeps a register of women who are happy to talk to you on the phone or in person. Some of the other organisations listed also offer counselling to patients and their families.

Groups of women who have had breast cancer have been formed at many hospitals; details will be available at your hospital or local library. CancerLink (see Useful addresses) has a list of self-help groups all over the UK. For some women, self-help groups are wonderful, a chance to get out of the house, meet other people and make new friends. In some ways, life is easier for women who return to work soon. Others return from hospital to an empty house, if they live alone – or they are left alone all day to brood while their husband or partner goes out to work.

'I cried buckets when I first came to the group,' Mandy said. 'At last I met women who had gone through the same thing and who could really understand how I felt. For the first time I could say whatever I liked without choosing my words so as not to upset anyone. I hadn't expected it would do me any good. I only came to the group because I was early for my clinic appointment, and the waiting room was crowded. Now I come every week.'

Elizabeth, who doesn't have breast cancer, complained jokingly about her friend, Marian. 'When we met for coffee, not only did she insist on going through her breast operation blow by blow, but she couldn't stop talking about the breast-cancer group at her hospital. You'd think it was a club the way she talks about it.'

Many women make new friends for life, and really look forward to their weekly meeting. Others find the meetings depressing, with everyone discussing their operations and their worries. Try going along and see how you feel yourself.

There is a move to form separate self-help groups for younger women whose concerns and problems are naturally somewhat different from those of older women, and there are also groups for women whose cancer has spread. If you are interested ask the breast-care nurse or get in touch with CancerLink (see Useful addresses).

Different responses

Women vary enormously in their response to finding out that they have breast cancer. You may suspect you have cancer because you have found a lump, or you have had a mammogram and been sent an appointment to attend hospital. You still have a little hope that, after all, you and the doctors are wrong – that it's a benign lump, or the wrong person's mammogram, or anything. Several women said their first reaction was relief that they finally knew the worst. Not knowing for certain was harder to bear.

Women's responses vary – and we may swing from one to another during diagnosis and treatment. Most of us have good days and bad days.

Fighting your cancer

There is some evidence that women who have a positive attitude, who say they won't give in, have the best chance of survival – though more research needs to be done in this area. These women want information about the various options and the likely outcomes. They are determined to face up to whatever comes.

Some of us get caught up in what has been called 'the prison of positive thinking'. Everyone tells us we've got to be positive and fight our cancer, but we all have negative feelings about our breast cancer. We must learn not only to be positive, but also to express our natural sadness, anxiety and anger. The important thing is for us to be able to acknowledge and express our feelings, whether positive or negative, and then go forward.

Denial

Some women simply reject the knowledge that they have breast cancer and refuse to face facts. They are quite likely to have delayed seeking advice when they first found a lump, and may not have attended for mammography. They try to pretend everything is fine even when they feel terrible, and just won't admit they have cancer. They may respond to having cancer by refusing to take an active part in decision-making, or to fight for survival, saying, 'What will be, will be.' They are convinced from the start that any treatment is a waste of time. There is some evidence that such patients have a worse chance of survival than those with a more realistic attitude.

Stoical response

Some women take their diagnosis in their stride with quiet acceptance, and maintain a philosophical attitude throughout their treatment. This should not make the rest of us (the majority) feel guilty or inadequate about our own feelings.

Anxiety and depression

Breast cancer is an anxious-making and depressing life event. Depending on their personality and the amount of support they get from family and friends, most women come to terms with their disease and take up their life again. Some, however, become seriously depressed. They need counselling and may require anti-depressant tablets. If you feel you are dwelling constantly on your cancer and that life seems to have lost its meaning, that nothing is enjoyable, don't wait. Go and see your doctor or contact the breast-care nurse and get help. Most of us think about our cancer often, but like ill-fated love affairs, we get over it in time, and are able to enjoy life again.

Taking control

Many women feel better about their cancer if they feel they have a measure of control over what happens to them. I was very happy to allow my doctors to decide on my initial treatment, but once that was over I firmly put myself back in the driving seat. Some women don't want to be involved in choosing their own treatment – and that's fine too. With all the emphasis on self-empowerment such women get to feel guilty. They shouldn't. Doctors have easy access to the latest information on the latest forms of treatment. If you want them to decide what's best for you, on the whole they will be delighted to do so.

Men with cancer

You might think that men wouldn't have the burden of worrying about their body image if they get breast cancer – but they do. They have the additional problem that breast cancer in men isn't a 'respectable' cancer. They may feel they can't talk about it at work or with their friends. Men have many of the same fears and personal problems as women have. While breast cancer tends to occur at an older age in men than in women, some younger men also develop it.

> Alec hated waiting in the breast clinic, the only man among 30 women. 'I always seem to get an appointment on a day when none of the women has brought a husband or male partner – and I feel a real prat on the beach with only one bosom. I don't like it when people stare at the side with the nipple missing and want to know the reason. If I say I had breast cancer they think I must be a transsexual or something. And it's not something I can talk about over a drink at the pub.'

BCC (see Useful addresses) can put you in touch with other men who have had breast cancer. They are very willing to talk about your problems, either in person or on the telephone.

13

Breast cancer and work

Help with housework

In an ideal world, a woman who has breast surgery would be able automatically to get help with cleaning, ironing, shopping and collecting children from school – but it's often not that easy. Ask to see someone from the Social Services Department at your hospital before you are discharged, and ask about a home-help. The provision of help is means-tested, so you will be asked to complete a financial assessment form and you may have to contribute a proportion of the cost. Your GP, social worker, care manager, or breast-care nurse completes a Full Community Care Assessment form, and you should be assessed within a week. There is now provision for boroughs to buy in home-help time from the private sector, though priority is given to people who need personal care with washing, dressing and so on.

Now is the time to ask for help from husbands, partners, neighbours and friends, until you have got back the full use of your arm and feel up to everyday tasks. Older daughters may understandably feel resentful if everyone assumes they will automatically take over.

Having time off work

You have no legal obligation to tell your employer exactly what is wrong, and you may prefer to be vague about the reason for your hospital appointment until the diagnosis is confirmed. Unless you have a special reason, it's best to tell someone in authority once you have a definite diagnosis. You can make it clear that it's in confidence and that you don't want a lot of sympathy from your fellow workers.

You will need a doctor's certificate if you are off work for more than seven days, and that will have your diagnosis on it.

When planning time off work for hospital appointments, always allow extra time for travelling and for waiting. People working in hospitals are aware that your time matters, but they also can't help feeling that their first priority is to do their job properly. If it takes more time, so be it.

Medical certificates

The Social Services Department at the hospital will be able to tell you all about the certificates you need – or you can ask the breast-care nurse, the ward sister or the oncology sister. For the first week you will need a self-certification form, on which you state you have been off sick. After seven days of sick leave your employers will want a medical certificate. If you wish, you can ask the personnel officer or your supervisor to keep the diagnosis to themselves.

Time off for hospital visits

If you have radiotherapy or chemotherapy, you will need time off work for your appointments. You are entitled to Incapacity Benefit (see below) for the days on which you have treatment. You may feel under the weather during the treatment, though perhaps able to go into work. Talk to the personnel manager when you feel up to it. They may be able to transfer you temporarily to lighter, less demanding work.

> Friends of ours are model employers who got upset when one of their staff with breast cancer didn't keep them informed. Theirs is a small firm and everyone counts. 'If only she would just let us know how things are going, whether she can come in even for a few hours a day. We could decide whether or not to get a temp', they said.

Claiming benefit

An account of the present situation (early 1996) is given here – but do remember that the rules governing benefit change without notice. Consult the Benefit Agency, your social worker, the breast-care nurse or a Citizens' Advice Bureau about the up-to-date situation. You should also consult leaflets IB201 and IB202 available at most post offices.

Statutory Sickness Pay and Incapacity Benefit

If you have paid enough National Insurance contributions and have a permanent contract with an employer, you can get Statutory Sickness Pay (SSP). It is payable if you are off work for four or more days in a row (including Sundays and Bank Holidays). It is not payable for the first three days, but thereafter it is paid to you by your employers for up to 28 weeks.

After that you normally get Incapacity Benefit, which has now replaced both Sickness Benefit and Invalidity Benefit. If you are on Unemployment Benefit you need to switch to Incapacity Benefit. Normally you have to be ill for four or more days together to get this benefit. If you have to go to the hospital for chemotherapy or radiotherapy, you can get benefit for the total number of days you attend, added together.

If you have not paid sufficient contributions, or are on a very low wage, you may still be entitled to Income Support and help with your council tax and housing costs. Extra benefit may be payable if you have children. Married women and widows who have paid reduced rate National Insurance contributions cannot normally claim Incapacity Benefit, but special rates apply to help some widows to qualify.

Disability Living Allowance and Attendance Allowance

If you are under 65 and need help with personal care or getting around, you could be entitled to Disability Living Allowance (DLA), which is a tax free benefit. To qualify for this you normally must have needed help for three months, and must be requiring it for a further six months or more.

Attendance Allowance (leaflet DS 702) is a tax-free benefit for people over 65 who need help with personal care. It does not depend on your having paid National Insurance contributions. To qualify for this you must normally have needed care for six months.

Special rules

Social workers are able to supply information on the various benefits which are available to patients who are terminally ill. Such patients normally have an automatic right to claim benefit, even if at the time they don't require nursing help. Claims are dealt with immediately, and there is no waiting period before the benefit is paid.

Invalid Care Allowance for your carer

The person who is looking after you, your carer, may be able to get Invalid Care Allowance if you are getting either Attendance Allowance or Disability Living Allowance at the middle or higher rate.

Getting help with forms

My friends in social services advise that patients ask advice on benefits while they are still in hospital.

> I arranged to be sent a number of leaflets on benefits, but I didn't find them at all easy to follow. Though they were clearly written, there seemed to be so many 'ifs' and 'buts', I would certainly have needed help with sorting out just what I was or wasn't entitled to.

The phone number of your local Benefits Agency will be in the telephone directory, or you can phone the Department of Social Security (DSS) freephone helpline (see Useful addresses). If necessary, the staff can go through the procedure with you step by step, and help you complete the forms.

Travel costs to hospital

This is a means-tested benefit for those who get Family Credit, Unemployment Benefit, are on Income Support or on a low income. You can get travel costs to and from hospital for treatment under the NHS as an in-patient or out-patient. It is important that you keep your tickets for proof of travel, and take evidence of being on benefit when claiming fares from the hospital cashier. Without them, you won't be reimbursed.

Free prescriptions

Women and men over 60 automatically get free prescriptions, and all medicines given to patients while they are in hospital are free. Any drugs given by drip, or medicines taken while you are being treated in hospital or in the oncology department, are free of charge. Medicines are also free if you or your partner get Income Support or Family Credit or are on a low income, if you are pregnant, or have had a baby within the previous 12 months. Full details are in leaflet P 11.

Everyone else has to pay for their medicines, so you should ask your doctor for the maximum number of tablets he is allowed to prescribe. Regardless of how many tablets of any one drug he prescribes, you pay one prescription cost. If you are likely to need more than five items in four months, or more than 14 items in a year, it works out cheaper to buy a season ticket.

Free hospital appliances

Post-mastectomy bras and breast-forms (prostheses) are free if you had your operation under the NHS. You should check the position concerning replacements when you see the hospital surgical appliance officer. You may require a temporary wig while having chemotherapy, though most women don't need one. Wigs are free if you are an in-patient when they are prescribed, or get Income Support or Family credit or are on a low income. Otherwise you have to pay a contribution towards their cost.

Citizens' Advice Bureaux

Citizens' Advice Bureaux (CAB) are staffed by people who have had training in a wide variety of common problems. In larger bureaux most of the staff are salaried, though in the smaller, suburban offices, more voluntary staff are used and only the manager will be paid. They know lots about the various benefits and types of help available. The atmosphere is friendly and highly professional. Look up their number in your local phone directory if you haven't got all the help you need from your hospital's social services department.

Extra financial help

You may find you incur extra costs after your treatment – such as heating, laundry and so on – or you may have lost or gained weight and need new clothes. Ask to see the social worker who can apply to certain charities on your behalf. Vouchers are available to obtain domestic appliances like washing machines and vacuum cleaners.

Going back to work

Some women want to go back to work as soon as possible, while others need longer. Give yourself plenty of time to recover. Many of us underestimate the upset of a major event like cancer, even when we've got over the initial shock.

> The surgeon looking after me threatened to chase me out if I returned to work at the hospital in less than a week. I promised to take a week off after my lumpectomy and axillary clearance, and went back to work the following Monday. I stayed at work for the subsequent couple of weeks before starting radiotherapy, and for the month of X-ray treatment. It was a mistake: I got very tired and depressed. It would have been more sensible to take a couple of months off. In the end I had to do that anyway.

Some women get over their operation very quickly, while others find that it takes months to feel fit again, even if everything went smoothly. It's easy to misjudge just how exhausted you will feel. Warn your employers that you will have to see how it goes. You may be surprised at just how understanding they are. It may be possible to change to part-time or a less demanding job for a bit. You don't have to feel guilty if you need to take off several months. Do what is right for you. Some women go back in weeks, others need six months.

Coping with colleagues

Expect to get very tired and even a bit weepy when you first go back to work. You may get upset that people seem to ignore you because they are too embarrassed to ask how you are. They are not sure whether you want to talk about your cancer, so they retreat into silence. Some women hate being fussed around and want to be treated as if nothing had happened. Others like to be coddled a bit. Just make up your mind what you want and tell one or two people. It will soon catch on. Don't be afraid to change your mind. You may like to be fussed around occasionally.

Margaret has a responsible position in a large organisation. 'I only told my supervisor and line manager,' she said. 'I didn't want to walk into a room and find that everyone had stopped talking because they'd been discussing me.'

Sarah decided to 'come out' and tell everyone. 'At first it was great,' she said, 'people fussing around me and being extra nice. But then I got fed up with people coming up all the time and asking how I was. I felt it was time to get on with my life.'

Betty said, 'Everyone was really lovely. I didn't know there were two other women in the firm who'd had breast cancer. Molly had the same surgeon. She thought he was very abrupt and crabby but, like me, she trusted him. It was like being in a new club. The other women were very supportive too.'

It can be worrying to be off while your work piles up. We all feel irreplaceable.

A very sensible nurse was blunt when I said, 'Who will cover for me while I am in hospital?' 'Suppose you'd had a heart attack or been run over by a bus.' she said. 'The department would have had to cope without you then.' She was right. They did cope – but I'm still not sure I was pleased to find I wasn't that important.

Sometimes fellow workers go on treating you like an invalid for too long.

June told me she used to get cross after she'd had her operation. She hated people coming up to her very confidentially and asking in a whisper how she was. 'But you look so well,' they would say, as if breast cancer should make you feel ill generally.

You just need to talk to the people around you and make the first move. Tell them if you want to talk about your cancer and everyone will be relieved to know where they stand.

Elizabeth was sick of people saying, 'I know how you must feel'. She felt no-one who hadn't had cancer, and hadn't had to face the reality of a breast being removed, could possibly know just how devastating it was, and how you could think of nothing else.

Giving up work

For some women, having breast cancer is the last straw and they feel finally they want to give up going to work. That's fine too. Take advice from your personnel officer or the social worker and sort out your pension.

I took early retirement, though not because of my breast cancer. Like all the other old 'biddies' I now wonder how I ever had time to go to work, what with my painting and art history and writing circle and cookery classes! I now have to look at my diary to see whether I can come to tea. Every day is full of things I enjoy and didn't have time for when I was working.

14

Secondary breast cancer

Unlike primary cancer of the brain, lungs or bowel, primary cancer of the breast causes no generalised symptoms. It doesn't make you feel ill, and doesn't by itself shorten your life. It is only if and when it spreads to vital organs like the liver, lungs or brain to form secondary cancers that it causes damage to your body as a whole.

No-one can be certain how long someone with secondary cancer will live. It could be months or it could be years. Drugs are available to help the symptoms, and however long you have can be rewarding and fulfilled. Many of us feel that, provided we are not in pain and we have a good quality of life, we'd like the extra months or even years. Even though there are no guarantees, we'd like to see a child through A levels or see our first grandchild.

> My particular research interest was in those substances cancers produce that help to distinguish one cancer from another. Many breast cancers, for example, make substances found in milk. Using special techniques, even secondary breast cancers in bone can be shown to do the same, and it is one way of finding out where a secondary cancer originally came from.
>
> Patients who have widespread cancer do not have the most rosy outlook. When I used to lecture about my work, I always said that, provided the quality of my life was good, I would do anything to have the extra time even if the treatment was unpleasant. Now that I have had breast cancer, I feel this even more strongly. I have a caring husband, four gorgeous grown-up children and one lovely grand-daughter. I'd like to live to see more grand-children, and my children all settled, happy and fulfilled.

Women who have had breast cancer have a dread of the cancer recurring – it can be devastating when you think you have been cured and the cancer returns. You may feel it's not worth having further treatment and that nothing is worthwhile. At present, it is not known whether secondary breast cancer can be cured – but what is known is that treatment, whether conventional or complementary, can improve the quality of your life. *You can add life to your years, if not years to your life.*

Some women who have been 'fighting' their cancer by strict diets, visualization and so on, feel guilty when their cancer recurs. If only they had tried a bit harder. Those around them may feel just as bad. If only they had been more supportive, cooked more of the correct foods. This is the down-side of taking control and is not based on any scientific evidence. Don't feel it's all your fault, neither your secondary cancer nor your primary one.

How do you know you have secondary cancer?

Some women constantly fear that they have secondary cancer, while others are able to put the thought out of their mind. Often, women with secondary cancer have no symptoms and don't realise they have secondary cancer until they go to hospital for a check-up. Some women with secondary cancer feel generally run down, more tired, and under the weather. If this is new for you, go and see your doctor – but remember that such feelings are common after surgery, and after a course of radiotherapy or chemotherapy, and usually do not indicate secondary cancer.

Spread to the bones, liver or lungs

Usually secondary breast tumours first appear in one organ – the liver, the lungs, the bones, or the brain – and less often in several sites. The appropriate treatment for each is different, so your treatment may be different from someone with secondary deposits in a different part of the body.

If breast cancer spreads to a bone it may cause an aching pain, or weaken the bone, so that quite a minor knock causes it to break. These fractures (called pathological fractures) often heal if an operation is carried out to fix the ends together with a metal pin or plate, and the fracture site is given radiotherapy. If you have a number of secondary cancers in your bones, calcium, the main constituent of bone, may seep into the blood-stream, causing you to feel tired, thirsty and ill. This can be detected by a blood test and treated.

Secondaries in the liver may make you feel tired and unwell, or you may notice your waist band is getting too tight. If the drainage of the bile produced by the liver is blocked by enlarged lymph glands, you may develop jaundice and the whites of your eyes and your skin become yellow and itchy. This may be helped by radiotherapy to the liver, or high doses of drugs called steroids.

Women with secondary cancer in their lungs may notice that they have a cough which they can't shake off, or they may find they get short of breath very easily. Sometimes the cancer cells attach to the covering of the lungs (the pleura), which reacts by producing fluid that makes you more breathless. This can be helped by draining off the fluid through a thin tube inserted in your side under a local anaesthetic.

If secondary cancers occur in the brain, they may make the pressure to build up, causing headaches or nausea. If they occur in a part of the brain which controls a specific function, you may notice that an arm or a leg becomes weaker or that you are more unsteady than usual.

Tests for secondary breast cancer

The tests the doctor orders to determine whether you have secondary cancer depend on where you have symptoms, but a blood test and chest X-ray will probably be first. One of the various scans described in Chapter 6 may be ordered.

Treatment of secondary breast cancer

All three types of medical treatment used for primary breast cancer – radiotherapy, chemotherapy and hormone therapy – have a place in the treatment of secondary breast cancer, and are more fully described in Chapter 9. You may be given one of the oestrogen-reducing drugs like Tamoxifen, aminoglutethamide, Lentaron or Zoladex, or other endocrine therapy. Less often your doctor may suggest removal of your ovaries to remove the source of oestrogen. Surgery otherwise has little place in secondary cancer, except to fix a fractured bone so that it can heal. Occasionally, if there is a single secondary cancer in the brain it can be removed and then the site treated by radiotherapy.

Palliative care

Palliative care is treatment which deals with the symptoms without aiming to cure. The term has come to have a doomsday ring about it, but in fact we are used to having palliative care for all sorts of things. When we have 'flu we take aspirin to help bring our fever down and treat our headache or backache, but we still have the illness, influenza, which must take its course.

The aim of palliative care is to improve the quality of life while avoiding treatments that make you feel bad – unless they have a real chance of affecting your cancer. It is not yet known whether high dose multi-drug chemotherapy and stem cell transplants (discussed in Chapter 9) will result in long term cure.

Treatment of pain

There are several drugs available to deal with pain at any site, or you may consider one of the complementary therapies like acupuncture. The Macmillan nurses (see Cancer Relief Macmillan Fund under Useful addresses) or nurses from your local hospice are particularly skilled in helping you to find the most suitable for you.

Complementary therapy

Some women seek complementary therapy (see Chapter 11) when they first find they have breast cancer, but it is mainly those who have secondary cancer who feel they want to see if there is something that will really cure them. Anyone who has tried relaxation, massage and some of the other therapies can vouch for how good they make you feel – and they can certainly improve the quality of your life. There is as yet no scientific evidence to show that they can help you live longer or can cure secondary cancer. If you do have a recurrence while following some form of complementary therapy, try not to allow yourself to feel guilty. It is not your fault. The best therapists will help you with this, but some may leave you feeling that, if only you had had more faith or stuck more rigidly to the diet, this would not have happened.

We have not yet begun to fathom the many ways in which we influence our body's behaviour, mind over matter. However, when you look at cancer cells under the microscope, watch them growing and dividing, it is hard to believe that the sheer belief that they will shrivel up and die will in fact make them do so. It is also impossible to believe that relaxing your diet, losing faith in any particular therapy, giving up control, will make them suddenly grow.

Self-help groups and counselling

Much is talked and written about famous people who fought their cancers to the end. Women who know they have widespread cancer often feel that they too must put a brave face on things. They don't have to. Certainly, it doesn't help to make everyone around you miserable, but you also owe something to yourself. Joining a group of women in the same situation allows you to cry and say how you really feel.

Some women feel better talking to someone in private, and counselling may be what helps them most. Several cancer charities keep registers of counsellors and self-help groups (see Useful addresses). There are now a few groups specially for those with secondary breast cancer.

When cancer is not held back

Just over 70% of women who develop breast cancer in the UK are over 55 years old, with most cases being diagnosed between 60 and 75. Many of those women will have a normal span of life, even though they have breast cancer. We all hope not to die of our disease, though some 38% of us will do so. It is easier for women like me who have reached retirement age, have had a satisfying career, with a lasting marriage, grown up children and grandchildren, to contemplate death with a degree of equanimity. We at least can feel we have had a fair crack of the whip. It is much harder for young women to contemplate the thought of death. They may have young children, just be contemplating a career move or generally have unfinished business.

The hospice movement

Hospices are places devoted to the care of those who do not have long to live. In hospices, people with terminal cancer are cared for in a dignified environment, if there are reasons why they do not wish to remain at home or it is not possible for them to do so. You can go into a hospice for a short period to give your family or the person caring for you a break.

Hospices have several facilities on offer. They include:

1. Short term stay in the hospice, either to give the family a chance to go on holiday or just for a rest (respite care), or to get symptoms, particularly pain, really well under control. Hospices are not designed for long term admission. It is easier to come to terms with the need for strong pain-killers like morphine in the caring, yet highly professional, atmosphere of a hospice.
2. Day-care, with visits of moderately well patients to the hospice for a variety of activities, outings, art therapy and so on.
3. Home-care to help control any symptoms, particularly pain, and to provide support for the patient and their family.
4. Counselling for families.

Hospices may be funded largely by charitable funds and partly or wholly by the local health authority, but all treatment is free. At first I was going to use the word 'institution' to describe a hospice, but this gives completely the wrong impression.

As part of the research for this book I arranged to visit two hospices near London. My image of a hospice was very negative, and I wanted to see for myself what they were like before mentioning them in this book. I imagined them to be rather like the geriatric ward I had worked in as a young house officer: dreary, full of sad old people waiting to die and smelling rather nasty.

They were absolutely nothing of the kind. If you had been told that these were small hospitals for heart patients or for those with any other non-cancer disease, I am sure you would have believed it. The atmosphere was bright and cheerful, with some single rooms, some small wards, day rooms, a canteen for visitors, and a day centre with an exhibition of patients' pottery and paintings. In both hospices I visited there was a tremendous feeling of commitment. Of course I hope not to need their services, but I certainly feel I could face a time in a hospice with equanimity.

Financial assistance

The social worker can give you information on benefits available to patients who are terminally ill. Special rules apply so you would automatically get the highest rate of Incapacity Benefit, and will be able to get one or more of the additional attendance allowances (see Chapter 13).

15

A more hopeful future?

Is it all doom and gloom?

The answer is 'No'. At least six out of ten women survive their breast cancer, and if we can pick up more cancers when they are small and less likely to have spread elsewhere we will do better still. With small cancers (less than two centimetres in diameter) survival reaches 84%. Research is being carried out in many centres worldwide into more accurate ways of diagnosing breast cancer and more effective methods of treating it. At the moment, the cause is unknown, but much work is going on to try to discover its cause or causes and how to prevent it. In this era when new information spreads so rapidly, progress in breast cancer research is known about very rapidly anywhere in the world.

It is depressing to think that little progress has been made in the treatment of breast cancer in the last 50 years in so far as survival is concerned, but finally the death-rate in the UK from breast cancer is falling. In Scandinavia, screening has reduced deaths from breast cancer by up to 40%. In the UK, the screening programme and increased Breast Awareness have begun to bring down the proportion of women who have advanced cancer when they first see a specialist. Early detection and removal before the cancer has spread is one approach, but others are being investigated. More emphasis is now placed on attempting to find the causes of breast cancer and prevent it.

New approaches

Advances are often sudden. For example, cancers of the testis, the commonest tumours in men aged 25–34 in the UK, were often fatal before the discovery of platinum-containing drugs. Now more than 85% of men with testicular cancer survive.

New and more powerful drugs are being found, and research into the genes involved in breast cancer may allow scientists to devise treatments aimed at combating gene defects. In other cancers, treatment with a powerful anti-cancer drug linked to an antibody to the tumour – the so-called 'magic bullet' – has proved useful. This approach might turn out to be suitable for breast cancer. Drugs which stop tumours from developing their own blood supply, so they shrivel away and die, may prove of value.

142

Efforts are being made to improve our body's fight against our cancer, by stimulating our immune system with drugs called 'biological response modifiers'.

If you have breast cancer, even if it has spread, hang in there. Tomorrow a miracle drug or some other type of therapy may be discovered which will revolutionize treatment.

Women are spear-heading efforts to make more funds available for research, particularly into prevention, but as long ago as 1896 the famous German pathologist, Virchow, said 'Indeed, a great deal of industrious work is being done and the microscope is extensively used, but someone needs to have another bright idea.' We could say the same today, one hundred years later.

Useful addresses

Sending for information

All of these organizations are charities, so if you wish to send for any of their booklets, please send a large stamped and addressed envelope. Contributions to their funds are always gratefully received. They are listed in alphabetical order.

BACUP (British Association of Cancer United Patients)

121–123 Charterhouse Street
London EC1M 6AA
Freephone: 0800 181199 (outside London)
Counselling service: 0171–696 9000 (London based)

BACUP was founded by Dr Vicky Clement-Jones following her own experiences as a patient with ovarian cancer. It provides nationwide information on cancer, by telephone and letter, as well as a one-to-one counselling service. BACUP produces an excellent series of booklets on the main types of cancer and kinds of treatment, and on living with cancer. The phone lines are very busy so be persistent and, if asked, leave a message. They do ring back.

Breakthrough Breast Cancer

103 Kingsway
London WC2B 6QX
Telephone: 0171–405 5111

This charity engages in collecting money for one particular research centre. It does not offer information or advice.

The Breast Care Campaign

1 St Mary Abbots Place
London W8 6LS
Telephone: 0171–371 1510

The Breast Care Campaign mainly deals with benign breast problems, but has a leaflet available on breast problems of all kinds.

Breast Cancer Care (BCC)
(previously the Breast Care and Mastectomy Association)

Kiln House
210 New King's Road
London SW6 4NZ
Nationwide freephone: 0500 245 345

13a Castle Terrace
Edinburgh EH1 2DP
Edinburgh helpline: 0131 221 0407

Suite 2/8
65 Bath Street
Glasgow G2 2BX
Glasgow helpline: 0141–353 0539

BCC was founded by Betty Westgate, herself a breast cancer patient, and provides advice and information. Volunteers who have had breast cancer are available for support on a one-to-one basis for men as well as women. People are accepted as counsellors only if at least two years have passed since their own surgery, and who have therefore come to terms with their own feelings. BCC produce several booklets on breast cancer. The organization also runs an excellent, personal prosthesis (breast-form) fitting service and give advice on suitable bras.

Cancer Research Campaign (CRC)

6–10 Cambridge Terrace
London NW1 4JL
Telephone: 0171–224 1333

All money donations are gratefully received, as is the donation of money or goods to one of the CRC shops. Leaflets on breast cancer are available, but are mainly intended for health professionals.

CancerLink

17 Britannia Street
London WC1X 9JN
London helpline: 0171 833 2451
Asian support line: 0171 713 7867
MAC line for young people: Freephone 0800 591 028

CancerLink was started in 1982 by two ex-cancer patients, Petra Griffiths and Ann Jenkinson, together with Val Box and Julian Gross. The organization provides a free and confidential service offering information and support on all aspects of cancer, by letter or telephone. It publishes a directory of cancer support and self-help groups in the UK, and produces a range of publications on breast cancer.

Cancer Relief Macmillan Fund (CRMF)

15–19 Britten Street
London SW3 3TZ
Telephone: 0171–351 7811

CRMF supports and develops services for people with cancer at every stage of their illness, and may be able to offer financial support. It funds the Macmillan Nurses whose services are available free of charge for home care and hospital support. It also supports Macmillan doctors, cancer care and information units. Together with the King's Fund it has recently produced a directory of breast-cancer services for GPs.

Citizens' Advice Bureaux (CAB)

National Association of Citizens' Advice Bureaux
115–123 Pentonville Road
London N1 9LZ
Telephone: 0171–833 2181

Local CAB addresses can be found in your phone directory

Free advice and help on many subjects, including social security benefits, family and personal matters.

Crossroads (Association of Care Attendant Schemes)
(England, Wales and Northern Ireland)

10 Regent Place
Rugby
Warwicks CV21 2PN
Telephone: 01788–573653

(Scotland)
24 George Square
Glasgow G2 1EG
Telephone: 0141–226 3793

National voluntary organization for Crossroad schemes which provide care attendants to come into the home to give the carer a break.

Department of Social Security (DSS)

You may already know where your local DSS office is. If not you will find the address in your local telephone directory.

Freephone: Social Security: 0800 666 555

Freephone: benefit enquiry line (BEL) 0800 88 22 00
Freephone advice in other languages:
Chinese: 0800 25 24 51
Punjabi: 0800 52 13 60
Urdu: 0800 28 91 88
Welsh: 0800 28 90 11

Freephone Health Information Service: 0800 66 55 44

Institute for Complementary Medicine

POB 194
London SE16 1QZ

Provides a list of complementary therapists. Send a large, stamped and addressed envelope and a note stating the information you require.

Lymphoedema Support Network

The Royal Marsden Hospital
Fulham Road
London SW3 6JJ

Contacts:
Sally Harrison 0171 433 3410
Helen Payne   0181–748 2403
Lucy Wolfe   0181 647 6456

Information, support and advice on lymphoedema.

Marie Curie Cancer Care

28 Belgrave Square
London WS1X 8QG
Telephone: 0171–235 3325

Runs eleven nursing homes throughout the UK, and a community nursing service to give extended care to cancer patients at home.

The National Cancer Alliance

POB 579
Oxford OX4 1LP
Telephone: 01865–793566

A relatively new alliance of patients and health professionals, their relatives and friends. Has published a Directory of Cancer Specialists in the UK.

The Patient Education Group

The Royal Marsden Hospital
Fulham Road
London SW3 6JJ
Telephone: 0171–352 8171

This group publishes a useful series of leaflets on various aspects of cancer. They may make a charge for them.

RAGE (Radiotherapy Action Group Exposure)

Joyce Pritchard
24 Edgeborough Way
Bromley
Kent BR1 2UA
Telephone: 0181–460 7476

Information for women who have pain or weakness in their arm following radiotherapy.

The UK National Breast Cancer Coalition

POB 8554
London SW8 2ZB
Telephone: 0171–720 0945

Launched in October 1995, the UK National Breast Cancer Coalition campaigns to ensure access for all to state-of-the-art treatment for breast cancer, for more government funds to be made available for research, and for breast cancer to be seen as a top priority in health care with women taking an influential role in decision-making. Membership is open to all whether as patient, partner, health professional or friend. Send a large S.A.E. for further information.

Women's Nationwide Cancer Control Campaign

Suna House
128–130 Curtain Road
London EC2A 3AR
Helpline: 0171–729 2229

Encourages measures for the prevention and early detection of cancer in women. Produces a wide range of leaflets and posters.

Regional Helplines

For full list contact CancerLink (address above).

Tak Tent

4th Floor
G Block
Western Infirmary
Glasgow G11 6NT
Telephone: 0141–334 6699

Provides information, counselling and support for cancer patients, relatives and professional staff involved in their care.

Tenovus Information Centre

142 Whitchurch Road
Cardiff CF4 3JN
Telephone: 01222–691998

Provides a counselling and information service personally or over the telephone.

The Ulster Cancer Foundation

40–42 Eglantine Avenue
Belfast BT6 6DX
Telephone: 01232–663439

Provides information over the phone on all aspects of cancer.

Further reading

Baum, M., Saunders, C., and Meredith, S., *Breast Cancer: A Guide for Every Woman*. Oxford University Press, 1994.
A concise factual book about breast cancer.

Batt, S., *Patient No More: The Politics of Breast Cancer*. Scarlet Press, 1994.
An intriguing book about male and female attitudes towards breast cancer and possible causes, written with a strong North American bias.

Edwards, B., *Drawing On The Right Side Of The Brain*. HarperCollins, 1993.
A book about drawing for everyone.

Fallowfield, L., and Clark, A. *Breast Cancer*. Routledge, 1992.
A book about the psychological aspects of breast cancer mainly for health professionals.

Faulder, C., *Breast Cancer and Breast Cancer Care*. Ward Lock, 1995.
Published in association with Breast Cancer Care (BCC).
A short, easy-to-read book on breast problems.

Love, S.M., with Lindsey, K., *Dr. Susan Love's Breast Book*. Addison-Wesley Publishing Company, Second Edition 1995.
Unfortunately, this is not on sale in the UK. A very complete account of breast problems from the American point of view, written sympathetically by a woman breast surgeon.

McConville, B., *Mixed Messages: Our Breasts In Our Lives*. Penguin, 1994.
A general survey of the social and medical aspects of breasts.

Stanway, A., *Complementary Medicine. A Guide To Natural Therapies*. Arkana Penguin, 1994.
A short, readable introduction to complementary medicine.

Glossary of medical terms

Alopoecia
Loss of hair

Adjuvant therapy
Medical treatment of cancer given in addition to surgery; if given before surgery it is called neo-adjuvant therapy.

ANDI
Aberrations of Normal Development and Involution. Another name for benign breast disease.

Anti-emetics
Drugs to prevent nausea and sickness, or to treat them.

Axilla
Armpit; underarm.

Axillary clearance
Removal of all of the lymph glands in the armpit.

Axillary sampling
Removal of some of the lymph glands in the armpit to see if they contain cancer.

Benign tumour
A tumour which grows by expansion, not by pushing out extensions into the surrounding tissue, and which does not spread elsewhere in the body. Only dangerous in very special circumstances, in the brain, for example.

Biopsy
Removing part of a lump to examine it under the microscope.

Blood count
Counting the number of red cells (required to provide enough oxygen for the tissues), white cells (required to fight infection), or platelets (required to avoid bleeding) in the blood.

Breast-form or 'falsie'
An artificial appliance (prosthesis) to pad out a bra to make the side which had a mastectomy or lumpectomy look like the other breast, when clothed or wearing a swimsuit or night-dress.

Carcinogen
Any substance, form of energy, or activity that can cause cancer.

Carcinoma
A cancer of cells which cover or line the body or internal organs, and of glands like the breast.

CIS (Carcinoma *in situ*)
The presence of very abnormal cancerous cells which have not yet broken out into the surrounding tissues.

CMF
Abbreviation for a commonly used combination of drugs used in the treatment of breast cancer – cyclophosphamide, methotrexate and 5-fluouracil.

CT Scan (Computerized Axial Tomography)
Set of X-rays which show a part of the body in imaginary slices.

Chemotherapy
Treatment with drugs which kill cancer cells (cytotoxic drugs).

Clavicle
Collar bone.

Cyst
Cavity (hole) in the tissues, usually containing fluid.

Cytologist or Cytopathologist
Doctor who examines cells removed by fine needle aspiration (FNA), or cells in fluids taken, for example, from breast cysts.

Cytotoxic drugs
Drugs which kill cancer cells.

Diagnosis
Finding out what's wrong with you.

DNA
Deoxyribonucleic acid – the material from which genes are made.

Drip
Fine tubing inserted into a vein – usually in your arm – for giving blood transfusions and a variety of medicines, particularly those which must be given over a long period.

Drugs
All medicines, tablets and potions are called 'drugs' by doctors. Used medically, the word does not only mean a drug of addiction.

Duct
A natural tube in the body like those along which eggs pass (the Fallopian tubes) or fluid is carried back from the tissues (lymphatic ducts).

Endocrine gland
Gland that produces a hormone.

ER
See Oestrogen receptor (Oestrogen is spelt 'estrogen' in the USA).

Five-year survival
This is usually given as a percentage and is the amount of people living after first diagnosis of their disease. Because nowadays people tend to move around the country (or countries), it is difficult to follow them up for more than five years and figures for longer periods become increasingly inaccurate.

FNA (Fine needle aspirate)
Taking cells from a lump (or enlarged lymph gland) by sucking them out (aspirating them) using a fine needle and hypodermic syringe. They are then examined under the microscope by a cytologist.

Hickman line
A special kind of drip in which a fine plastic tube is inserted into a large vein at the root of the neck. It is left in place and can be attached to a tiny pump which delivers drugs over a period of time. It avoids repeated drips into your arm.

Hormone
Also called a chemical messenger. Substance produced by an endocrine gland. It is discharged into the blood-stream and so reaches other parts of the body.

Hypothalamus
A part of the brain that controls the pituitary gland, and also produces antidiuretic hormone, which is important in maintaining our water balance, and oxytocin which is important in labour.

Immune system
A vital body system which protects us against infection and cancer. It is composed of antibodies, which circulate in the blood and are produced by our plasma cells, and a variety of cells, which each have a special protective function – some against infections, some against cancer. If our

immune system is depressed, or deficient for any reason, we are more likely to develop infections – and cancer. Anti-cancer drugs themselves depress immunity; care must be taken to avoid infection while they are being used.

Incidence
Number of new cases of a disease per annum. Because there are different numbers of people in each age group, the Office of Population, Censuses and Surveys (OPCS) corrects incidence rates (given as number per 100,000 population) accordingly – there are always less 90-year olds than 19-year olds. These figures are termed 'age-adjusted'.

Interval cancers
Breast cancers which come to the notice of the patient or her GP within the three-year gap which presently exists in the UK (1996) between invitations for mammography in the over 50s.

Lesion
A defect in any part of the body, from a scratch to a cancer.

Lobule
The part of the breast in which milk is produced.

Lumpectomy
Removal of the breast-cancer lump, along with a rim of normal tissue, leaving the rest of the breast intact.

Lymph gland or lymph node
Bean-shaped, tiny structure, important in immunity against infection and cancer.

Lymphatics
Fine tubes (ducts) though which fluid in the tissues passes back to the blood stream.

Lymphoedema
Swelling (oedema) of a part of the body due to damage to lymphatic ducts, or failure to form them properly. The pooled fluid (lymph) acts as an irritant and causes scar tissue to form, so unless treated early the swelling can become permanent.

Malignant tumour
A cancer. A tumour which grows into surrounding tissues, and which can spread elsewhere in the body.

Mammogram
A mammogram is a special type of X-ray which instead of showing only

the bones (and teeth) allows the soft tissues of the breast to be seen. Cancers (and normal breast tissue) show up as white structures against the darkness of the surrounding fat.

Mammography
The taking and interpreting of mammograms.

Mastectomy
Removal of the whole breast.

Metastasis
Secondary tumour which has spread to a site at some distance from the primary cancer.

Milk line
An imaginary line stretching from the armpit over the breasts to the groin. In some people additional nipples or breasts are found somewhere along this line.

Mitotic index
Except for eggs and sperm, human cells divide in half by a process called mitosis. When a part of the body or a cancer is growing, mitoses can be seen under the microscope. The number is the mitotic index. The faster a tumour is growing, the higher the mitotic index, and generally the more malignant it is.

Mortality
The number of deaths per annum for a group of people with or without a specific disease. Like incidence rates (see Incidence above), mortality rates (number of deaths per 100,000 population) are usually age-adjusted.

MRI Scan (Magnetic Resonance Imaging)
Takes a picture of your internal structure by passing you though a magnetic field and detecting the difference between tumours and normal structures.

Nausea
Feeling sick.

NK Cells
Natural Killer cells. Cells present in the blood and tissues which kill tumour cells, as well as dealing with some infections.

Neoplasm
A tumour. Usually refers to a malignant tumour.

NHS
National Health Service.

Node status
Whether or not cancer has spread to your lymph nodes.

Oestrogen (spelt estrogen in the USA)
The female sex hormone produced by the ovary throughout the menstrual cycle. Can also be produced in the body by conversion from male sex hormones and adrenal hormones, mainly in fatty tissue. Thought to be the most important factor in the development of breast cancer.

Oestrogen receptor (ER)
Molecules in cells which allow them to respond to oestrogen coming to them. Cancers with high levels of oestrogen receptors need oestrogen to survive and grow.

Oestrogen window
The time between the first development of the breasts at puberty and their maturity, when they are still very sensitive to high, potentially cancer-inducing (carcinogenic) levels of oestrogen in the body.

Oncogene
Genes thought to cause cancer. Now considered to be abnormal forms of naturally-occurring genes.

Oncologist
Doctor who treats cancer.

Osteoporosis
Thinning of bone. The commonest cause is age, and it is held at bay in women by their sex hormones. It therefore gets worse after the menopause.

Palliative care
Treatment to deal with symptoms; not aimed at cure.

Pancreas
Gland situated between the liver and stomach, which produces insulin among other substances.

Pathological fracture
Fracture (break) through a bone already weakened, for example, by cancer.

Pathologist
Doctor who examines tissues under the microscope and carries out post-mortems.

Pituitary gland
Very important, small gland at the base of the brain. Produces hormones that control the thyroid, adrenal, ovary and testes, as well as producing growth hormone and prolactin. It stores hormones from the hypothalamus.

Placebo
A substance made to look like a medicine but without any medicinal action. Given in controlled trials to half the patients to be sure the active drug, which is given to the others, is really working, not just making them feel better because they are under treatment.

Plastic (or cosmetic) surgery
Surgery aimed at improving your appearance. Also used for the very skilled surgery required to correct certain congenital defects – a cleft palate for example.

Ploidy
The number of sets of chromosomes in a cell. Normal cells are diploid – they contain two sets of chromosomes, one from each parent; eggs and sperm are haploid, they contain a single set each, which will merge in the new baby. Cancer cells are least aggressive when they are near to normal (diploid), and most malignant when they have all different numbers of chromosomes (aneuploid).

Prevalence
Number of people alive who have, or have had, a disease (such as breast cancer) at any one time.

Primary breast cancer
The original tumour in your breast.

Progesterone
Female sex hormone produced by the ovaries in the second half of the menstrual cycle. Helps prepare the womb for reception of a fertilised egg. Necessary for development of lobules in the breast.

Prognosis
What is likely to happen to your disease.

Prophylaxis
Doing something to prevent a disease, like immunisation against measles, mumps and whooping cough, or breast removal before cancer develops in women from high risk cancer families.

Prosthesis
An artificial replacement for part of the body. Dentures, hip joints and breast-forms are all prostheses.

Radiotherapy
Treatment with high energy beams, most often X-rays.

Recurrence
Cancer that comes back in, or very close to, the original site.

Regression (of tumours)
Getting smaller or disappearing altogether.

Secondary cancer
Spread of cancer to a site separate from the primary cancer.

Side-effect
Unwanted, usually unpleasant, effect of some drug or treatment.

Sign
Something detectable by a doctor or X-ray or other test.

Stem cells
Primitive cells from which mature cells develop.

Sternum
Breast-bone.

Symptom
Something a patient experiences.

Ulcerate
Break through the overlying skin (or bowel, or bladder etc).

Tamoxifen
The best known anti-oestrogen drug.

TDLU (Terminal Duct Lobular Unit)
The breast duct and its milk-producing lobules. The part of the breast from which breast cancers are thought to develop.

Therapy
Treatment.

TNM classification
An international classification based on Tumour size, Node status and the presence or absence of Metastases.

Tumour

An abnormal growth of cells forming a lump (mass).

Tumour suppressor genes

Genes in cells which stop them from becoming malignant. They often also act as normal growth control genes.

Ultrasound

A method of examining the body by picking up distortion in transmitted sound waves too high to be heard by the human ear.

Index